Fighting Cancer
with More than Medicine

To Chris who helped to "build" Macmillan

[signature]

Fighting Cancer
with More than Medicine

A HISTORY OF
MACMILLAN CANCER SUPPORT

PAUL N. ROSSI

The
History
Press

First published 2009

The History Press
The Mill, Brimscombe Port
Stroud, Gloucestershire, GL5 2QG
www.thehistorypress.co.uk

British Library Cataloguing in Publication Data.
A catalogue record for this book is available from the British Library.

ISBN 978 0 7524 4844 2

Typesetting and origination by The History Press
Printed in Great Britain

Contents

Acknowledgements

I would like to thank Richard Hambro, Douglas Scott, Nick Young, Joan Bebbington, Derek Spooner, Ann Rogers, Simon Henderson, Jean Gaffin and Jacqui Pugh for all the help and encouragement they gave me in writing this book. Mostly, I want to thank my wife Lynne for living with the project for several years and for always giving me honest and objective advice.

Sadly, Richard Hambro and Derek Spooner died before this book was published. It serves as some small memorial for all they did to help people with cancer.

Any errors of fact or interpretation are mine alone.

Paul N. Rossi
London

Foreword

This is a remarkable story of a group of people, led by one person, who changed the way in which cancer care is delivered in the United Kingdom. With a vision, and enormous enthusiasm and determination, Douglas Macmillan and subsequently millions of others saw a better way forward, and they achieved their vision. They realised that to care for patients and their families with cancer required more than medicine, drugs, radiotherapy and surgery. They saw very clearly that care, compassion and education were of the utmost importance.

The story begins at the very start of the twentieth century in 1911 and progresses from the provision of information and lectures, to fund raising and the provision of unique services and of 'Macmillan Nurses' by the end of the century. It is a social history as well as one concerned with the relief of suffering. There is a history of medicine here too, as the various forms of treatment and provision of services, including the beginning of the NHS are described. The inter-relation between the various charities is also developed fully.

There were three aspects that particularly struck me. The first was the enormous determination of people who want to change things for the better. There are setbacks and obstacles, but they are all overcome and as the momentum grows, more and more people realise what this really means and get behind it. It becomes an enormous social movement. The power of that movement for change becomes unstoppable. Douglas Macmillan could rightly be proud of his achievements, but also I suspect surprised at just how successful it was.

The second aspect which was relevant was the power of the non-medical aspects of care. I have written elsewhere that the aim of medicine should be to assist healing. By this I meant that healing is a process which makes people whole. Medicines and surgery can do much, but improving quality of life is more than that, it requires a different approach and one which recognises the needs and wishes of individuals. Macmillan's ability to bring that healing, and to provide relief in tangible ways, is one of the most remarkable parts of the story.

My third aspect was more personal. I have been connected with Macmillan for almost forty years. I have seen at first hand what can be achieved. My own involvement in Macmillan and in other patient support groups made me recognise just what a source of skill and expertise lies in patients and their families. I am sure I am not alone in realising that this was one of the most powerful learning experiences in my professional career.

However, I am also part of the Clan Macmillan and am proud of its motto 'Miseris Succurerre Disco' – I learn to look after those in need. What a wonderful motto for a clan and a cancer charity. It says it all: learning by doing, putting into practice the best ideas, and at the same time directing efforts to those in need; it summaries for me what Macmillan is all about and why it has been so successful in changing the lives of people with cancer for the better.

I wish it continuing success.

Professor Sir Kenneth Calman, KCB, DL, MD, FRCP, FRCS, FRSE

I

A Disease Comes of Age

The National Society for the Prevention and Relief of Cancer, as today's charity Macmillan Cancer Support was first known, was founded in the closing years of Edwardian England. This is much earlier than is often thought, probably because the Macmillan name has only been widely used for the last thirty years or so. However, of the better known cancer charities of modern times only one, the Imperial Cancer Research Fund, founded in 1902, is older.[1] The Cancer Research Campaign was established in 1923, and Marie Curie Cancer Care in 1948. The Leukaemia Research Fund was founded in 1962. Those cancer charities which focus on one or more specific cancers, such as breast cancer, bowel cancer, prostate cancer or lung cancer, were all started relatively recently. One feature of cancer research and cancer care, particularly in the latter part of the twentieth century, has been a big expansion of the number of charitable organisations dedicated to fighting the disease, or to caring for its patients, or both. Today, the Charity Commission for England and Wales has many hundreds of cancer charities on its register, and the registering authorities in Scotland and in Northern

Ireland many more. There is no part of health care in the UK that is more vibrant or more motivated than the cancer sector. One hundred years ago, the picture was quite different.

The Society, with its origins in 1911, was borne out of the growing horror of cancer and the impact that it was having on people's lives, and out of the sheer despair that so little could apparently be done. The Society was quite different from what had gone before. Its emphasis was not on research, but on prevention and relief, and most particularly at the beginning, on prevention. It was a society of volunteers, and it was a society of lay people not dominated by the professions of medicine or science. This made it unusual, and possibly unique, amongst disease fighting organisations of the time. But it was also an organisation very much in keeping with its times. In the Victorian period, cancer had become recognised as one of the great challenges to human health and happiness, and with the new century came the hope, and also the confidence, that the disease could, at last, be overcome. The nature and the causes of cancer had become a common topic for speculation and discussion amongst doctors and public alike, for now the illness was touching so many people. In 1901, maybe with the experience of his own family in mind, King Edward VII issued a challenge to doctors and scientists with the words:

> There is still one … terrible disease which has, up to now, baffled the
> scientific and medical men of the world, and that is cancer. God grant
> that before long you may be able to find a cure for it, or check it in its
> course …[2]

In the year following, a joint committee of the Royal College of Physicians and the Royal College of Surgeons founded the Cancer Research Fund, later granted by the king the prefix 'Imperial'. The launch of the new charity came in the form of a letter to *The Times* signed by sixteen eminent people from medicine, science and public life appealing for funds. So important was this cause of cancer research regarded, that Arthur Balfour, the prime minister, signed the letter and presided at the Fund's first annual general meeting. The Prince of Wales regularly attended subsequent annual meetings until he became King

George V in 1910. In its first year, over £50,000 had been donated to the charity, while the prime minister lamented that it had not been more. In his mind may well have been the words of some of the founders of this new endeavour, that cancer was 'an obscure disease' and that the research would probably 'extend over a considerable number of years'.[3]

This opinion did little more than reflect the realisation that any conclusive knowledge about cancer was elusive and that there were many theories and ideas about its nature and its causes, which were often in conflict. Distinguished men of medicine and science, and amateur epidemiologists too, had been theorising about the causes of cancer for decades. Some believed that a bacterium or some other parasite was responsible for the malady, often after observing the similarity between the progressive deterioration and wasting that came in the late stages of cancer with that of tuberculosis. Others blamed a changing diet and implicated all sorts of foodstuffs from frozen meats to tomatoes. There was a debate about whether residential buildings could harbour cancer, passing it to each occupier in turn, and sales of the disinfectant Izal were promoted as one way of destroying the cancer-causing agent, whatever it might be. One member of the Court of Common Council of the City of London, Mr Elliott, blamed cancer on living conditions and told his council colleagues in 1852 that this 'dreadful disease is engendered in the low and filthy habitations of the poor, and that the corporation has in its power the means of prevention, however difficult might be the means of cure'.

Ladies were warned not to clean their ears with pins because the metallic elements were thought to be carcinogenic. One piece of research purported to show that cancer occurred only in coal burning areas and never in places that burned peat, and so concluded that sulphur must be the deadly substance causing the disease.[4] Rather less spurious research at the Middlesex Hospital demonstrated a hereditary link in some cancers. The potential danger of recurrent irritation as a carcinogen had been known about since Dr Percival Potts of St Bartholomew's Hospital in London recognised scrotal cancer in chimney sweeps as long before as 1775, and this led others to reason that some trauma, such as a blow, could be the causal factor of other cancers. However, there was still dispute about whether cancer began as a local condition before spreading to other parts of the body, or whether it was some underlying body-wide ailment which then manifested itself in local eruptions of tumour. When Arthur Mayo Robson, a distinguished surgeon and vice president of the Royal College of Surgeons, said in 1904 that, 'Of the true cause of cancer we really know nothing', he was not far from the truth.[5]

Cancer was not of course some new illness to hit the nineteenth and early twentieth centuries. It is as old as life itself. Cancers can be identified in the bones of dinosaurs and evidence of malignant disease has been found in the examination of mummies from Egypt and Peru. Indeed, the first written descriptions of cancer appear on ancient Egyptian papyri written 3,500 or more years ago. The Edwin Smith papyrus, one of the earliest known tracts on the treatment of disease and named after the American who purchased the document in Cairo in 1862, gives both a diagnosis and a rather gloomy prognosis for breast cancer. The classic translation reads:

> If thou examinist a man having bulging tumors on his breast, and if thou puttst thy hand upon his breast upon these tumors, and if thou findst them cool, there being no fever at all when thy hand touchest him, they have no granulation, they form no fluid, and they are bulging to thy hand. Thou shouldst say concerning him: One having bulging tumors. An ailment with which I will not contend.

The Greek physician Hippocrates, writing in the fourth century BC, is credited with giving cancer its name. The word 'cancer' derives from the Greek word *karkinos*, which means crab, and which is thought to have described the physical appearance of an advanced cancer of the breast. Hippocrates also wrote about the symptoms of bowel cancer, of skin cancer, and of many other conditions which could well have had a malignant cause. His Roman colleague, Aulus Cornelius Celsus, also wrote about the disease and depressingly recorded in his encyclopaedia that, even after surgical removal, cancers always re-appeared. But if the Greeks and Romans were keen observers of the disease, their understanding of biology was primitive. They believed that the body had four fluids or four humours that, in balance, were vital for health.

The fluids were blood, phlegm, yellow bile and black bile. Cancer, they thought, was caused by some imbalance of the humours and, in particular, an excess of black bile probably brought about by some form of immoderate living.

These hypotheses, postulated by the second-century Greek physician Galen, were accepted science for 1,500 years. Usefully, they were not incongruent with the Christian view during the Dark and Middle Ages that illness and disease were brought about by the wrath of God as punishment for sin. St Bernard, the founder of the Cistercian Order, forbade his monks from studying medicine, believing that the only remedy for illness and disease was prayer, and Pope Innocent III made a similar pronouncement in 1139. Where treatment of malignant disease was available, then in common with the treatment for other ailments, it tended to be limited to the ancient practices of blood letting, cupping, primitive surgery and the taking of various potions. *The Leech Book of Bald,*[6] a treatise on medicine from Anglo-Saxon times, refers to some bizarre and unwholesome treatments for the wounds sometimes associated with cancer, while also acknowledging the often incurable nature of the disease:

> Burn a fresh hound's head to ashes, apply to the wound. If it will not yield to that, take a man's dung, dry it thoroughly, rub to dust, apply it. If with this thou art not able to cure him, thou mayst never do it by any means.

Interestingly, it is known that some ancient practitioners used as cancer treatments a range of plant extracts that are known to have anti-carcinogenic properties, but the grim likelihood of the outcome was clear. In fact, cancer is not much referred to in the writings of these times. Although exist it certainly did, it is impossible to quantify in terms of numbers, age distribution or geographical occurrence. Human health was dominated instead by catastrophic outbreaks of plague, leprosy, smallpox, measles, cholera and other infectious diseases. These diseases, together with accidents and famine, ensured that most people died when they were comparatively young. Cancers had little time to develop. So, while physicians, barber surgeons and apothecaries did see cases of cancer, and particularly those cancers which had some external manifestation, the number would likely have been very small. On the other hand, wise or experienced opinion from the ancient Egyptians onwards was that cancer was almost always incurable.

The texts of medical learning from Hippocrates onward may accurately describe the appearance and manifestations of a few cancers, but rarely do they describe adequately, if at all, the suffering that those with cancer had to endure. This is perhaps not so surprising, given the suffering that accompanied so much of the human condition in those times. The pain and death of cancer probably ranked little differently from the pain and death that was associated with so much of life. Moreover, the Christian view that illness and disease was God's punishment, often led those concerned with spiritual matters to believe that some pain and suffering prior to death was a blessing if the soul was to be saved. In fact, medical men would have little to do with patients whose condition was hopeless or who were dying. This was the reserve of the clergy. The notion of a good death, particularly in the Catholic tradition, lay not in minimising a patient's suffering at the end of life, but in praying for redemption and resisting temptation to the last.

Some centuries pass before writings adequately try to explain what cancer meant to those unlucky enough to be afflicted with the disease. Richard Wiseman,[7] Sergeant-Chirurgeon to King Charles II, described how he treated a patient with a cancer in the mouth. The surgery consisted of burning away much of the gums and palate with red-hot iron instruments. The treatment was so unbearable that it had to be carried out over three days and, not surprisingly, the patient later died. Wiseman knew that his surgery was not likely to be successful and his work was criticised as unethical by contemporaries, but he wrote to stoutly defend his practice:

> These unsuccessful attempts may render us extream cruel to those who feel not the misery of those poor creatures (who) suffer with cancers of their mouths … eating and gnawing at the flesh, nerves and bones … which rendered them unable to swallow and to eat and drink. Death is their only desire (that drives them) to try a doubtful remedy.

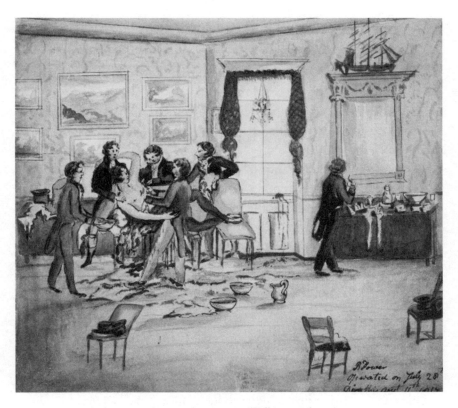

Cancer surgery before anaesthesia and antisepsis. (Wellcome Library)

In other words, so terrible was this malady that patients would try any treatment that gave even the smallest glimmer of hope, even though excruciatingly painful. Another surgeon, John Brown,[8] movingly described the examination of a woman with breast cancer while he was a clinical assistant at the Minto House Hospital in Lanarkshire:

[She] sat down, undid her gown ... and without a word showed me her right breast. I looked at it and examined it carefully ... What could I say ? There it was, that had once been so soft, so shapely, so white, so gracious and bountiful, so full of blessed conditions, – hard as a stone, the centre of horrid pain, making that pale face, with its grey, lucid, reasonable eyes, and its sweet resolved mouth, express the full measure of suffering ... Why was that gentle, modest, sweet woman, clean and lovable, condemned by God to bear such a burden?

Brown goes on to say that the following day, 'my master, the surgeon, examined [the patient]. There was no doubt it must kill her, and soon. It could be removed – it might never return – it would give her speedy relief – and she should have it done.'

The patient was indeed operated on, and endured, without anaesthesia, slow and painful surgery, but she died some days later as a result of an infection in the wound.

Accounts of the sufferings of people with cancer can also be seen in contemporary press reports. One example is from *The Times* on 16 October 1801. It reported the death of the Countess of Holderness:

> On Tuesday afternoon, died at her house in Hertford Street, Park Lane ...
> at the advanced age of seventy six. Her Ladyship's complaint was a cancer
> in the mouth, which had destroyed the upper jaw, and part of the tongue.
> The original cause of this dreadful malady was a cancer in the left breast,
> which had increased to such an alarming degree as to render amputation
> necessary about three years since: and though at such an advanced age,
> her Ladyship bore the painful operation with uncommon fortitude, and
> concealed the knowledge of it from her grand-children. ... Her death is
> rather a consolation than a regret to her family, as she had been wholly
> nourished by suction for many weeks past.

The countess's amputation came as well before the invention of anaesthesia. For the less wealthy classes of society of course, surgery would have been out of the question. The disease would have taken its course, most probably without any treatment at all. Another report, from 9 March 1832, concerned a gentleman farmer from Salisbury, named Mr Bowles, who 'had been afflicted ... with a cancer in his face, which of late had destroyed his nose and a greater part of his face and mouth, and the entirety of his palate'. Such a ghastly manifestation of disease can hardly be imagined.

Twenty years later the suffering of Ada, Lady Lovelace, the daughter of Byron and an outstanding mathematician, was recorded in her diaries and of those who cared for her. She had a gynaecological cancer which progressed over two or three years, and ended with a terminal stage that lasted several months. According to her friend Mary Somerville,[9]

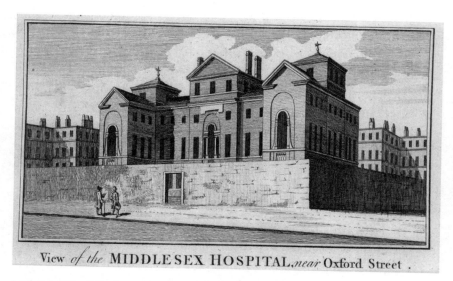

View *of the* MIDDLESEX HOSPITAL, *near* Oxford Street .

Middlesex Hospital where the first dedicated ward for cancer patients was opened in 1792. (Wellcome Library)

'I never heard of anyone who suffered such protracted intolerable agony'. Ada herself said that her pain was 'indescribable'. Periods of relative comfort could only be assured with larger and larger doses of laudanum,[10] until the pain became so overwhelming that only a chloroform-induced stupor could give her any relief. She died, terribly, at the age of 37. Others who described their own illnesses included the actor David Garrick,[11] who wrote just before he died at the age of 61 that, 'I have lost legs, arms, belly, cheeks and have scarce anything left but bones and a pair of dark, lack-lustre eyes that are retired an inch or two more in their sockets'.

The sufferings of people with cancer moved others to philanthropy and to a search for any means of bringing some comfort to those afflicted with the disease. In 1792 a gift from the brewer, Samuel Whitbread, paid for the first ever hospital ward solely dedicated to patients with cancer to be opened at the Middlesex Hospital in London. Patients were to be allowed to remain there 'until relieved by art or released by death'. A ward of twelve beds was endowed, together with an out-patients clinic. Cancer attracted the attention of the Society for Bettering the Condition and Increasing the Comforts of the Poor. The Society, founded in 1796 by, amongst others, the anti-slave trade campaigner

William Wilberforce, aimed to improve the welfare and condition of the common people.[12] In 1801 it announced its decision to fund a new cancer charity, the Institute for Investigating the Nature and Cure of Cancer. The most distinguished medical men of the time served on the cancer institute's medical committee, including Matthew Baillee, a physician to King George III, the surgeon Sir Everard Home, Thomas Denman the obstetrician, and John Abernethy, who would later be responsible for founding the medical school at St Bartholomew's Hospital. According to Denman:

> In the long train of diseases to which human nature is subject, no one is attended with more hopeless misery than that which is denominated cancer, whatever part of the body may be the seat of it. This occurs more frequently than is generally supposed; and a calamity so pitiable as that of persons afflicted with cancer, in any rank or situation in life it is hardly possible to imagine; their suffering being aggravated by the present insufficiency of medicine to afford any proportionate relief.

The committee planned to research the causes and the nature of cancer, but its work was short-lived because funding ran out. The lack of sufficient funds for medical research was not only a problem of recent times.

The first hospital to be dedicated to the care of cancer patients was The Cancer Hospital (Free), now the internationally renowned Royal Marsden Hospital in Chelsea. It was founded by Dr William Marsden in 1852. Marsden, who some years earlier had founded what is now the Royal Free Hospital in Hampstead, was a man of great compassion with a particular concern for the sick who were also poor. In 1846 his wife Elizabeth died of an internal cancer. Neither he, nor any of the other eminent doctors he consulted, could offer any treatment or hope before she succumbed to the progressive emaciation and weakness of the cancer's terminal stages. Moved by this experience, Marsden founded his cancer hospital for 'poor persons afflicted by cancerous conditions' and from its beginnings care was provided free of charge. Marsden freely admitted that medicine knew absolutely nothing about the disease and after the hospital had been open for a year, Marsden reported that: 'We have before us a wide and almost appalling sphere for

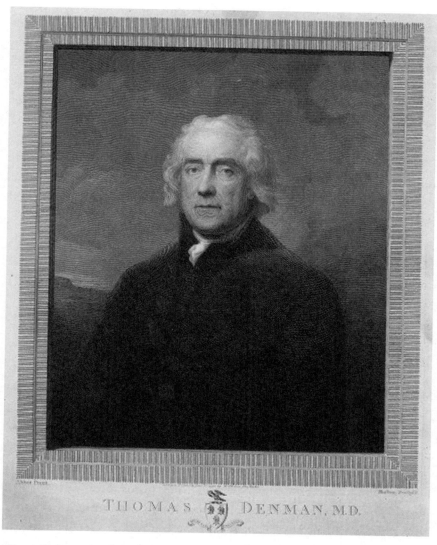

Thomas Denman, who said there was no more *hopeless misery* than cancer.
(Wellcome Library)

our exertions, humbling us by the present aspect of the extent to which
this disease is rife.'

Similar great foundations followed. The surgeon James Smeaton
Smythe founded the Liverpool Hospital for Cancer and Diseases of
the Skin in 1862. Glasgow got its own cancer hospital in 1886 when
the Glasgow Skin and Cancer Institute was founded, later called the

Beatson Hospital after Sir George Beatson, its first director of cancer services. Five years later the cancer hospital was opened in Manchester, funded by the estate of the industrialist Sir Joseph Whitworth. Richard Christie was an executor of Whitworth's will. He had a passionate concern for the plight of people with cancer and was the prime mover of the initiative. The hospital was later re-named in his honour, the Christie Hospital.

The growth of hospitals and clinics specialising in cancer was underpinned by a growing quest to understand the nature of the disease. As early as 1791, the physicians at the Manchester Infirmary announced that,

> We have agreed to keep an exact account of each case of cancer which shall come under our care; in which will be recorded a faithful history of the disease with its attendant circumstances and the effects of medicines and operations when necessary, together with the collateral helps to be gained by an enquiry into constitutional habits and diseases not strictly cancerous but probably connected to it. [13]

Scientific knowledge about the biology of cancer did indeed improve radically in the late eighteenth and nineteenth centuries, chiefly as a result of major advances in the studies of anatomy and pathology. The invention of the microscope allowed for the most intricate study of organs and the cells that build them. The British surgeon, Sir Everard Home, first described cancer under the microscope in 1830, and shortly afterwards, the French physician Joseph Récamier discovered how cancers spread to other parts of the body. The German doctor Rudolf Virchow described the integrated cellular construction of the body and founded the study of cell pathology. These scientists, and others, realised from their observations that cancer cells were quite unlike normal body cells. They were mutations growing out of control. Added to these micro-studies, by the middle of the nineteenth century, most of the common cancers of the internal organs, such as stomach, bowel, bladder, pancreas and oesophagus, had been described from post mortem examinations. Increasingly physicians were able to identify cancers from clinical symptoms. In a little more than 100

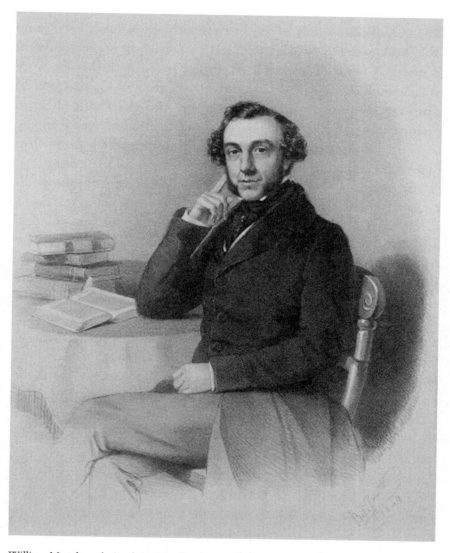

William Marsden admitted that medicine knew *absolutely nothing* about cancer. (Wellcome Library)

years, remarkably, more about cancer biology had been discovered than in the previous 2,000.

There were other world-changing discoveries during the Victorian years that brought about great strides in the treatment of cancer, or at least in cancer surgery which was the mainstream treatment then available. Surgery had always been an appalling prospect for a patient.

The unspeakable agony of the surgeon's knife was made even more diabolical by the knowledge that death followed the surgery, as often as not, as a result of infection. All this changed with the discovery of anaesthesia in the 1840s, and the introduction by Joseph Lister of antisepsis through his carbolic acid spray in 1870. These advances permitted longer and deeper surgical procedures, without pain and without risk of infection. Internal cancers became operable for the first time, and much more complex surgical procedures became possible.

The pioneer German surgeon Christian Billroth first performed a resection of the oesophagus in 1871, a complete excision of the larynx in 1873 and partial gastrectomy in 1881. American William Halstead introduced the radical mastectomy in 1891, and Scotland's Sir George Beatson introduced oophorectomy, the surgical removal of an ovary. Edouard Quénu of France began the removal of sections of cancerous bowel in the 1890s. For many malignant conditions, so long as the cancer was discovered in its very early stages, a full cure by surgery became possible for the first time ever. This was potentially an earth-moving step forward in treatment. Unfortunately though, cancers were rarely discovered so early in their development, and surgery was all too often only a palliative. The cancer returned within a year or two.

The closing years of the century brought further great leaps forward. In 1896 the German Wilhelm Röntgen, Professor of Physics at the University of Wurzburg, took medicine to a new horizon when he discovered X-rays. At first the magical rays could disclose only bones, but soon they were refined to show internal organs as well. X-rays would provide, of course, an invaluable aid to the diagnosis of cancer and to the work of the surgeon. Just as astonishing, however, experiments carried out on patients in the United States and in Europe showed that when they were exposed to X-rays tumours receded. This opened the way for radiotherapy, a revolutionary new cancer treatment.

Röntgen's work was followed two years later by the discovery of radium by Pierre and Marie Curie. Pierre showed that the radioactive waves from radium were even more effective in destroying cancer cells than X-rays, and these rays could be delivered by a phial of the radioactive substance inserted into the tumour as well as externally. From Vienna came the news that a man who had undergone several operations for

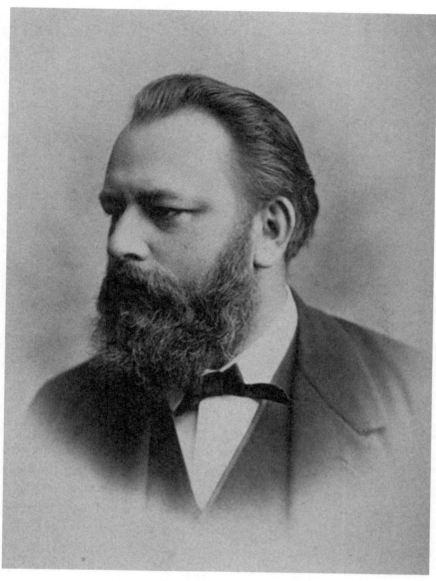

Christian Billroth – pioneer of cancer surgery. (Wellcome Library)

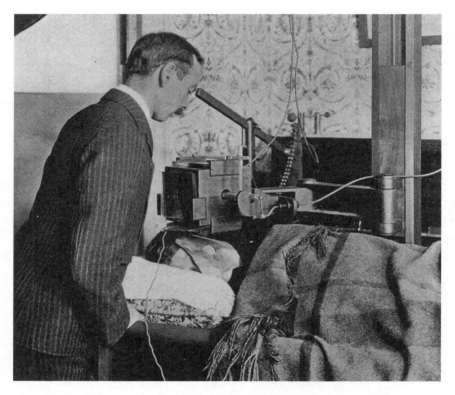

The early use of X-rays to destroy cancer cells. (Wellcome Library)

cancer of the lip and palate, and who was regarded as a hopeless case, had been cured by a strong application of rays from radioactive bromide. Other clinicians reported the cure of other face and skin cancers and the palliation at least of deeper-seated cancers. King Edward VII himself was a beneficiary of the new radium treatment when it was used to destroy a rodent ulcer on his cheek. There was excitement that cancer could become curable without the need for surgery at all. It was an incredible breakthrough.

The paradox for the time was that despite these great advances in medical science and technology, more and more people seemed to be suffering from, and dying from, malignant disease. This was not only the public perspective; it was supported by the statistical evidence. Compulsory registration of all deaths in England and Wales had been introduced in 1837 (and in Scotland and Ireland in 1851), and a doctor's certificate of each death and its causes was required by law from 1871. Statistics on the causes of death were collected and collated each year by the Registrars General. The crude figures showed a marked upward trend of cancer deaths throughout Queen Victoria's reign. In 1840 the number of deaths attributed to cancer in England and Wales was 2,786, or 17.7 of every 1,000 deaths. Fifty years later, the number of cancer-certified deaths was 19,433, or 67.6 of every 1,000 deaths. In other words, the number of cancer deaths as a proportion of all deaths had increased almost threefold.[14] As diseases like smallpox, cholera and typhoid began to recede into history, a new disease, in many ways more horrible, was coming into prominence. It began to affect more and more families.

To give the experience of just one family: by 1901, King Edward VII had seen the death of his maternal grandmother from cancer; lost a younger brother, Alfred, to cancer of the tongue; lost his elder sister, Victoria, to breast cancer; and she had lost her husband Friedrich, the German emperor, to cancer of the throat.[15]

The king's call to action, directed to the medical and scientific communities, doubtless reflected his deep and personal experience of the ravages of cancer and his commitment to do what was necessary to defeat this disease. But it was the experience of cancer in another family, and a similar commitment of one of its sons, that brought into being the charity which is the subject of this book.

Notes & References

1. The Imperial Cancer Research Fund merged with the Cancer Research Campaign in 2001 to become Cancer Research UK.
2. Speech to the International Congress on Tuberculosis held in London in July 1901.
3. See letter to *The Times* of 19 April 1902 from Adeline, Duchess of Bedford and others.
4. *The Cancer Problem, a Statistical Study*, by Charles E. Green, published by William Green & Co, 1911.
5. The Bradshaw Lecture, delivered at the Royal College on 1 December 1904.
6. *The Leech Book of Bald* is the oldest surviving English medical book. It was

written *c.* 930 in the reign of King Alfred. Leech is from the word *laece* meaning healer.

7. Richard Wiseman (1625–86) made his name as an army surgeon and became an expert in treating the wounds of battle.

8. John Brown (1810–62) wrote of his experiences as a surgical student in his book *Rob and his Friends.* The master referred to in the text was Dr James Syne, one of the greatest surgeons of his day. Brown's daughter married Joseph Lister.

9. Quoted in *Death in the Victorian Family* by Pat Lalland, published by Oxford University Press, 1996.

10. A concoction of opium and alcohol mixed in water.

11. 1717–79.

12. Founded in the middle of the Revolutionary and Napoleonic Wars with France, the society's founders hoped that improving the lot of the labouring classes would make them less amenable to radical ideas.

13. See *Portrait of a Hospital 1752–1948* by William Brockbank, published in 1952 by William Heinemann Ltd.

14. For a very good account of public health in the nineteenth century see *The People's Health*, by F.B. Smith, published by Croom Helm, 1979.

15. The liberal-minded Emperor Friedrich III died just three months after succeeding to the throne in 1888. His death marked the accession of his bellicose son Kaiser Wilhelm II. It is for speculation how different the history of the twentieth century might have been had cancer not struck when and where it did.

2

Foundation and Failure

The first charity dedicated to preventing cancer and to bringing relief to those with the disease was founded by Douglas Macmillan, with the support of his wife Margaret and a few friends and sympathisers. Macmillan, despite his distinctly Scottish name, was from Castle Cary, a small town in the eastern corner of Somerset. Douglas's paternal grandfather John was a draper from Ayrshire, who moved to Somerset and settled in Wincanton. Douglas's father, William, who would be the catalyst of it all, was born there in 1844. William married Emily White from Gillingham, in the neighbouring county of Dorset, and they moved to Castle Cary. William became a manager in the local horse hair-weaving business. He was a pillar of the local community. Elected to the parish council and the school board, he was also appointed a county alderman and a justice of the peace. Politically, he was the backbone of the town's Liberal Party, and in tune with the temperance tradition of the time he was proud to be a Good Templar.[1] William Macmillan was also, as to be expected, a stalwart of the local church – in his case the Congregationalist chapel. He was the head of a pious household.

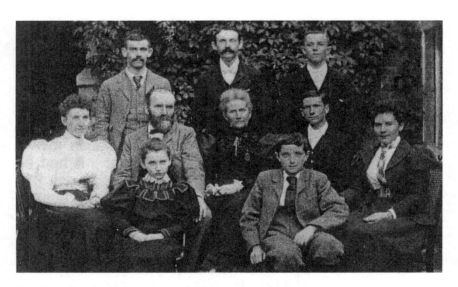

The Macmillan family. Douglas, aged about 10, sits at the front.

William and Emily Macmillan had five sons and three daughters; three of the sons would join the clergy.

Douglas was the seventh child, born on 10 August 1884. He first attended the local school and then became a boarder at Sidcot School at Winscombe in the Mendip Hills. Sidcot, a Quaker foundation, dates from 1699. It was, and still is, a school which values in its students not only academic success, but also a respect for the dignity and well being of others. The school's Quaker ethos lays stress on education being 'a joyful experience of self development and an inspiring introduction to the wonders of creation'.[2] Douglas became Sidcot's head boy in 1900, so he must have impressed his schoolmasters with conduct and endeavour that lived up to Sidcot's Quaker tradition. In 1901 he went to study at the Birkbeck Library & Scientific Institute, now Birkbeck College, in London. In 1905 he was appointed to a position at the Board of Agriculture and Fisheries, as the government ministry was then known, and he remained a civil servant until he retired forty years later at the age of 61. He became a specialist in public health and was elected a member of the Royal Institute of Public Health and Hygiene, and a member of the Institute of Statistics. Although Douglas Macmillan would spend most of his life in the London area (he moved back to Castle Cary in

1964), his affection for his Somerset home remained with him always, and so did a love of the countryside and of 'the wonders of creation'. He was a poet and storyteller, ever maintaining an interest in Somerset folklore and antiquities, and often using the pen name Douglas Cary. He published his works and those of his fellow Somersetians through the Somerset Folk Press, his own minor publishing house set up for the purpose. Macmillan is remembered as a very gentle, kind, quiet and unassuming man.[3]

Macmillan was twice married. His first wife, Margaret Miller, whom he married in 1908, was from Stonehaven in Scotland, and was sixteen years his senior. She had a profound influence on her young husband who left his father's Congregationalists for her Strict and Particular Baptism. Margaret died of cancer in 1957, but after having been successfully treated for the disease some thirty years earlier. A year later, Macmillan married his second wife, Nora Owen. She would outlive him, and she re-married after his death to become Mrs Percy Hill. She died as recently as January 2004 in Castle Cary. Neither of the marriages produced children. Both Margaret and Nora were to be strong supporters of the Society and to play an important part in its affairs.

The Strict and Particular Baptists were (and still are) an evangelical Christian sect with a belief that the words of the Bible are the authoritative words of God. Of special importance is their belief that salvation will not come to all, but only to a few, and that redemption as one of the few can only come about by living as God intended. Inspired by his new religion, but still with a good infusion of Quakerism, Macmillan set about spreading his message. In 1911 be began to publish a monthly magazine called *The Better Quest*, described as a journal 'devoted to truth and humaneness'. Its editorial and articles, often penned by Macmillan, were exhortations to think about God, the teachings of the Bible, and the relationship of man to God's creation. They lamented a society he saw as drifting away from the Christian ideal and becoming less, rather than more, civilised. The magazine was strongly committed to the kind treatment of animals and advertised meetings of the Christian Humane League held at the Macmillans' house. In March 1911 Macmillan wrote an article called 'In Cancer's Clutch', in which with considerable zealotry he declared that 'cancer is the fault of sin'. He quoted several

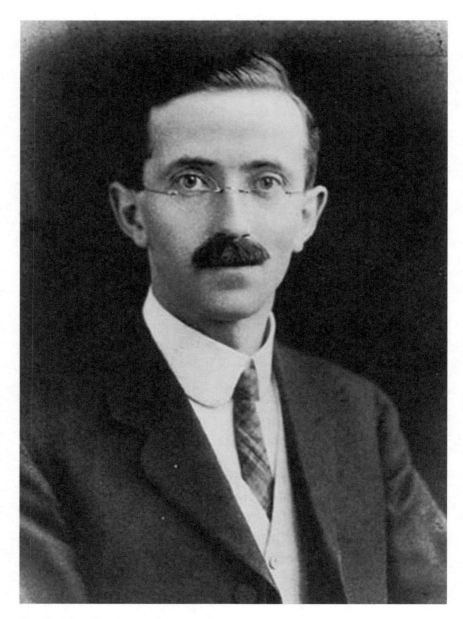

Douglas Macmillan as a young man.

medical authorities, including Dr Robert Bell, of which more later, who believed that diet, and particularly too much meat, was the root cause of cancer. Macmillan used as his argument for a vegetarian way of life, not surprisingly, a quotation from the first chapter of the Book of Genesis, 'And God said, Behold I have given you every herb bearing seed which is up on the face of the earth; and every tree in the which is the fruit of a tree yielding seed, to you it shall be meat'.

Macmillan could not have aired his forthright views on the causes of cancer at a less sensitive or appropriate time for, on 1 July 1911, Macmillan's father died of cancer of the oesophagus, ten days after surgery that was expected to extend his life by two or three years. He was 67 years old. This family loss had an enormous impact on Douglas. He explained that the death was the first break 'in a large and united family' and he described his father as 'the finest man I have ever known'.[4] The August edition of *The Better Quest* devoted three of its pages to William Macmillan's obituary, with the title page fully taken up with the exalted man's photograph. It was as if some national public hero had died rather than a small town civic notable, albeit a very worthy one. The young Macmillan had no doubt that his readers would be as woeful as he about his father's death. This sense of catastrophe, but also possibly guilt, drove the 27-year-old Douglas to commit the next fifty-three years of his life to preventing cancer or, more practically, to improving the lives of people with the disease. In Macmillan's own, rather understating words, 'the end came suddenly, and the tragedy of it so impressed [me] that a keen interest in the possibilities of prevention or amelioration in similar circumstances immediately followed'.[5]

A few days before William Macmillan's death, Douglas had received from him a birthday gift of £10. Douglas made this his first donation to 'fight the cancer scourge'.[6] He had set about founding the charity which now bears his name.[7]

Douglas Macmillan did not come to this challenge without many preconceptions, some of which had already been given some airing in *The Better Quest*. He believed that good health was linked to Godliness and, moreover, to his own interpretation of Godliness. He was certainly no follower of the medical establishment, and his words from the time show not only his lack of faith in conventional cancer treatments but also

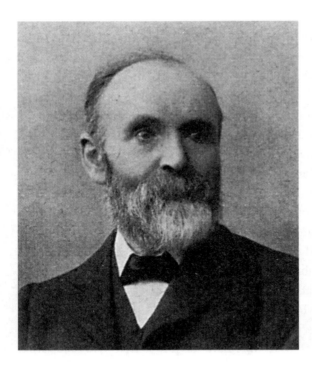

William Macmillan: 'the finest man I have ever known.'

a passionate belief in alternative theories. In the first leaflet he produced for his new charity, distributed in spring 1912, he explained that the Society had been founded because of two *facts*, which were nevertheless strenuously denied by medical and surgical orthodoxy. According to Macmillan these two facts were first, that the cause of cancer was *definitely known*, and second, that the *one reasonable and reliable treatment* was *also known*. Such certainty, unsupported by any evidence, is almost breathtaking. It was certainly more strident than wise. At best it reflects the faith and enthusiasm of a young and impressionable man, but it also shows a good degree of naivety. Macmillan's deeply held religious and moral convictions, which had made him a vegetarian, had convinced him also that eating meat must be the cause of this terrible malady. With these views it followed logically that Macmillan would also be utterly opposed to any form of scientific experimentation on animals.

The anti-vivisection movement was strong in late Victorian and Edwardian times, and at one point even Queen Victoria had expressed her sympathy for the cause (she wrote to the famous surgeon Lord Lister urging him to stop the use of live animals in research). The controversy was bitter, with many leading figures of the time taking one side or the other. Large-scale public demonstrations were held by The Animal Defence and Anti-Vivisection Society and addressed by eminent people of the day. George Bernard Shaw was a favoured speaker for the cause. In 1911 an anti-vivisectionist march from the Embankment to Hyde Park attracted thousands of supporters. Meanwhile, the Research Defence Society was set up by doctors and scientists to organise opposition to the anti-vivisection cause. Medical students joined the fray by violently breaking up anti-vivisection meetings and even demonstrating outside the Anti-Vivisection Hospital that had been founded in Battersea. There was real and genuine concern in the scientific community that medical research would be brought to a halt. This highly controversial subject was not just a division between scientists earnestly searching for cures to disease, and the idealistic or sentimental. It was then, as it is today, a clash of sophisticated moral arguments.

The case for the use of animals in experimentation was not helped in these times by the truths that much vivisection was undertaken for demonstration purposes and not research, and without anaesthesia, and that cats and dogs were most frequently the subjects of the practice. Nor was the argument helped by the arrogance of many leading doctors who rejected outright any restriction or controls on their activities. At the same time, there had always been a strand of medical opinion that was against vivisection for ethical reasons, or because of doubts that the information so discovered could be relevant to human biology. There were well-known doctors who joined the debate for the anti-vivisection cause. The book *The Shambles of Science,* by medical student and Swedish countess Louise Lind af Hageby, which exposed in a graphic and candid way vivisection at University College, London, had a considerable influence when it was published in 1903.[8] Macmillan was always ready to remind his friends that the great John Abernethy was a lover of animals and would never undertake vivisection of a living creature. Macmillan was determined that his new society would be for people who shared his moral philosophy and in the Society's first circular, Macmillan declared that the new organisation 'had no connection or any sympathy whatever with existing systems of Cancer Research, the representatives of which appear to be persuaded that "research" means "vivisection" ...'

The first constitution of the Society included a very clear statement of the fundamental beliefs that prospective members would need to hold. These were:

a) that the cause or causes of the disease may be more successfully sought by a careful investigation of the dietetic and other habits of the community than in the vivisecting laboratory,

b) that the treatment and cure of the disease may be more confidently looked for in the intelligent application of dietetic principles and the skill of the physician than in the surgeon's knife and the operating theatre *and*

c) that the prevention of the disease can only be secured by studying, and, where necessary, reforming the common habits of the community.

With such robustness, there could be no doubt whatsoever about where the Society stood on one of the most controversial issues of the day. It would also restrict the potential membership of the Society and set it in a position of antagonism towards the medical establishment.

The National Society for the Prevention and Relief of Cancer held its first Annual General Meeting on 12 December 1912. It was held in Douglas and Margaret Macmillan's home, 15 Ranelagh Road, off Lupus Street in Belgravia. The three-storey Georgian terraced house still stands, and today it bears a commemorative plaque to Douglas Macmillan. It is not recorded how many people attended the society's first meetings and the first annual general meeting, but given the size of the rooms in the house, it cannot have been many. The first months of the Society were important ones. Macmillan was busy putting together the structure of the organisation and finding like-minded people who were prepared to take on formal roles and positions. All of Macmillan's upbringing and education directed that his Society had to be a proper and upright organisation.

The chairman of the society elected in 1912 was Charles Forward. Aged 48 at the time, he managed the family bookbinding business and was a well-known writer about animal welfare, health and vegetarianism. Like Macmillan, he too believed that good health and a long life were the outcomes of healthy living of which diet was critical, and the avoidance

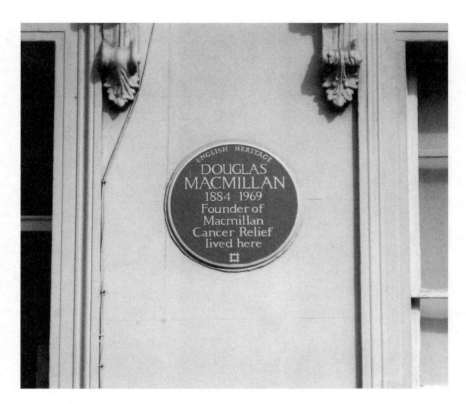

The commemorative plaque at 15 Ranelagh Road.

of meat the most important element. He was a leading member of the Vegetarian Society and published vegetarian cookery books, as well as serious works which often challenged the medical orthodoxy of the day. One of his books, *The Fruit of the Tree*, argued that illness and disease were the result of the modern-day diet because it had shifted so far from man's primitive, and therefore natural, diet. This strand of opinion, with several variations, was unconventional but not uncommon. The London physician Forbes Ross was a leading proponent of the theory. In 1912 he wrote *Cancer: its genesis and treatment*, in which he argued that it was modern food production that was the underlying cause of cancer. He postulated that potassium salts were essential to normal cell life and that these salts were too easily lost in food processing. He observed that his typical patient with cancer would eat rich and spicy foods, mostly meat; he would eat few vegetables and he would never drink the water

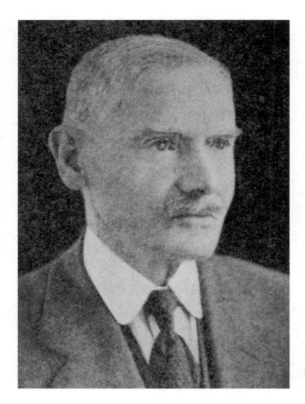

Charles Forward: vegetarian,
animal welfare campaigner
and Society vice chairman.
(The Vegetarian Society)

in which the vegetables were cooked. By contrast, in the Empire, Ross noted that healthy primitive peoples who ate fresh and raw foods, less meat and more vegetables suffered little cancer. Unfortunately, Ross was not taken seriously by many of his peers. In 1920 Dr John Murray, director of the Imperial Cancer Research Fund, rejected research into Ross's theories with the simplistically logical but quite absurd argument that cancers had been discovered in cows despite their being vegetarian.[9] Charles Forward nevertheless continued to proselytise the vegetarian case, and he played a major role in the Society until his death at the age of 70 in 1934.

The treasurer elected at the 1912 Annual General Meeting was William Wilsher, who held the post until 1931. Other members of the Society's governing council elected[10] included Margaret Macmillan, who had nursed her own mother through terminal cancer; John Proudfoot, a clothing manufacturer; the poet and critic, and sometime

Liberal Party candidate, Mackenzie Bell; Sir Frederic Cardew, former governor of Sierra Leone; and Lister-taught surgeon and medical director of the Battersea Anti-Vivisection Hospital, Dr Robert Bell. The last was also invited to become president of the Society. He was an obvious choice. Bell had just won an action for libel against Dr Ernest Bashford, the first director of the Imperial Cancer Research Fund, and the British Medical Association for an article that appeared in the *British Medical Journal* in which Bashford accused Bell of being a quack. Bell believed that all cancers were caused by some disorder of the blood and that surgery could never be an effective cure. Unless the underlying blood malady was tackled, he believed, the cancer would just recur, and Bell claimed he could diagnose cancer by microscopic examination of the blood. Bell blamed the underlying disease of the blood on diet, particularly too much meat and over-cooked vegetables, and irregular bowel habits. In support of his argument Bell, like Forbes Ross, drew attention to the low incidence of cancer in the under-developed world, and he too recommended a vegetarian diet. Bashford may well have been right to be critical of Bell's blood hypothesis, which was not based upon sound science, but a charlatan Bell was not. The view of the libel jury was that Bashford's polemic went much too far, and Bell was awarded damages of £2,000 (about £120,000 today).[11] As it turned out, however, Bell was not an easy colleague and his association with the Society was a short one.

Macmillan saw the importance of attracting to the Society people of standing and influence so long, of course, as they were people who shared his views and principles. He persuaded the Duchess of Hamilton to become the Society's first patron. The young wife of the 13th duke, the duchess was also a well-known campaigner for animal welfare. The list of vice presidents included Lord Charles Beresford, celebrated sailor and friend of the late king; Mrs Bramwell Booth, the Salvationist; Walter Crane, a well-known artist and Marxist; Roy Horniman, the actor, playwright, and later film producer; Sir George Kekewich MP, former president of the Board of Education and leading anti-vivisectionist; and Sir John Kirk, doctor, naturalist, explorer, and one-time assistant to David Livingstone. Among the medical practitioners elected were Dr Fergie Woods, who practised at the London Homeopathic Hospital;

Dr Charles Reinhardt, medical writer on diet and health; and Dr Joseph Stenson Hooker, another anti-vivisectionist who wrote critically of the direction of medicine at the time. Most significantly, the heroine of the anti-vivisection movement, Louise Lind af Hageby, became a vice president. The list of distinguished people, twenty-three of them in all, was impressive for a newly formed society with no track record to speak of. More importantly, it emphasised again the position of the Society in the Edwardian world as resolutely way out of step with the medical and scientific establishment.

The Society's register shows that in 1912 it had forty-four members, who each paid a minimum fee every year of 2s. 6d. (about £7.50 today). Douglas Macmillan had membership number one, and Margaret number 2. Like the Society's founders, the members were predominantly from southern England. Other donors numbered at about eighty, and together, subscriptions and donations amounted to £91. 9s. 6d. in the year to 31 December 1913. Total income for that year, including sales of literature and the Society's first legacy, was £187. 1s. 00d. (about £11,500 today). This was a modest sum indeed compared with the funds going to cancer research and it would not sustain a wide programme of activity. On the other hand, the Society did have one important benefactor who would help it through many years of financial famine. This was Margaret Macmillan. She owned property, and she was prepared to use income generated from rents to keep the Society afloat.

The two years before the outbreak of the First World War were busy and quite productive for the new charity. The Society's first objective, according to its constitution was to promote 'such conditions of living as shall secure the ultimate prevention of malignant disease'. Macmillan and his colleagues wasted no time before they started to spread knowledge and information about cancer – its causes, its symptoms, its treatments, and advice about prevention to the Society's members, and more widely to the public. This activity embroiled the Society in some of the heated discussions of the times about cancer, if only at the fringe. A series of five pamphlets, all but one written by Macmillan, were published in a collection called *The Crusade Series*. The first, written by Bell, was called *The Prevention and Relief of Cancer*, and it repeated his by now well-known theory of the causes of cancer. The paradox of the writings of Bell, and of Ross, Forward and Macmillan, is that while their science of cancer and cancer development might have been flawed, the preventative regime they recommended is an efficacious one. A diet low in animal fats and rich in fruits, nuts and vegetables, with the latter served uncooked or with light cooking to preserve the vitamin content, is exactly the diet recommended today as health giving and protective against cancer. The arguments and conclusions of the Society's pioneers, crude though they were, had more sense and logic than they have ever been given credit for. They were in the right ballpark all along.

The second *Crusade* pamphlet was called *The Tea Habit in Relation to Cancer*. It summarised a view, quite common at the time, even in conventional medical circles, that stimulants were a cause of cancer. The reasoning of the argument was that stimulants caused inflammation, and there was an established link between chronic inflammation and malignancy. Since tea contained the stimulants caffeine and tannic acid, Macmillan argued it ranked with alcohol, tobacco and meat as likely to cause cancer. Macmillan believed that such 'vices' should be abandoned if 'men and women [want to] become truly civilised'. The fourth pamphlet in the series, *On the Use of Violet Leaves*, was a review of how the leaves of violet plants were used, in various forms, to treat cancers and it called for further research into the subject.

It is easy to review these second and fourth tracts nearly 100 years later and to criticise them for having no real scientific merit. However, to be fair, they do no more than visit cul-de-sacs that many others, including medical practitioners, were also visiting. At the time, the paucity of knowledge about the causes of cancer was close to absolute. It is worth drawing attention to the irony that few contemporary authorities were making any link between smoking and cancer. On the contrary, cancers of the mouth were curiously often blamed on the irritation and soreness caused by broken pipes rather than the noxious clouds that flowed from them. It was not for another forty years that all medical opinion would agree about the direct causal relationship between tobacco smoke and cancer.

The third *Crusade* pamphlet was the most significant and would have the greatest impact. Published in 1913, it was entitled *The Cancer Mortality Statistics of England & Wales 1851–1910*. Known as the 'blue book', because of the colour of its cover, the publication was a comprehensive compilation of both aggregate and county-based statistics of cancer mortality over some sixty years. In this, Macmillan was in his familiar territory of public health and statistics. The significance of the paper was threefold. First, Macmillan demonstrated that deaths from cancer had increased from 497 for every one million people living in 1881, to 960 for every one million people living in 1910 – a rise of 93 per cent. Macmillan threw himself into the debate about whether the increase in the cancer death rate was real or illusory.

That the number of deaths recorded from cancer was increasing was beyond doubt. However, there was a strong line of argument, put forward by Sir Arthur Newsholme, Medical Officer to the Local Government Board, and echoed by Bashford of the Imperial Cancer Research Fund, that the crude statistics were misleading. They said that the apparent increase in the number of cancer deaths was really the result of better diagnosis. Deaths from cancer, particularly from cancers of the deep, internal organs, they suggested, had more frequently in the past been attributed to other causes. It is certainly true that death certificates of the nineteenth century often attributed death to age and debility, atrophy, marasmus, mortification and other vague conditions, many of which could well have been brought about by cancer. It was also well known that doctors were sometimes reluctant to speak of cancer even when they were sure that this was what they were dealing with – something that lasted well into the twentieth century.

As an example, in 1864 *The Lancet* reported that a doctor in Greenwich had certified the death of a patient to be due to neuralgia and phthisis (tuberculosis), although the doctor knew the patient had actually been suffering from cancer of the uterus. The doctor thought the real diagnosis too shocking to tell the deceased's relatives.[12] Of course, the extent to which the growth in the number of cancer deaths was real or illusory – and in truth there were elements of both – was important in understanding the epidemiology of the disease. But in terms of it being a challenge to public health and public well-being it mattered rather less. Whatever the underlying reason for the statistics, they represented substantial illness and suffering caused by cancer, and that was what Macmillan wanted to draw attention to.

Macmillan's second point compared the trend in cancer deaths with those from consumption, as tuberculosis was then more commonly known, and this was a theme that he would return to again and again over the next thirty years. Tuberculosis was a major killer in the nineteenth century. Macmillan showed that in 1860, for every 100 deaths from consumption, there were sixteen from cancer, but that in 1910, deaths from cancer had increased six-fold. Projecting these figures into the future he said:

> in five years time cancer will have outstripped its rival and will have a heavier death toll than consumption ... the one moreover is a conquered and dying foe; the other shows a prime vitality and rides rough-shod over the whole realm of medical ingenuity.

Deaths from tuberculosis were indeed falling rapidly, chiefly because of better standards of housing and public health in the towns and cities. Yet despite this, local authorities were being encouraged to provide more hospital facilities for patients with TB, and in 1911 tuberculosis even became a notifiable disease.[13] The Society decided not to campaign to make cancer notifiable, recognising that it was quite different in nature to infectious diseases. However, Macmillan was able to demonstrate just how inadequate hospital facilities were for patients with cancer.

The third issue raised in the pamphlet was the disparity of the cancer death rate between one county of England and Wales and another. Macmillan's analysis included a county map, shaded to show different death rates from cancer. It was reproduced for an article in *The Times* on 14 April 1914. Cancer hotspots were Huntingdonshire in England, and the counties of Anglesey, Merionethshire and Cardiganshire in Wales. The lowest rates of death from cancer were in the north-east and the north-west of England, the Midlands and south Wales (almost exactly the opposite of the distribution of cancer death rates today). The figures were puzzling. As Macmillan said in his introduction to the statistics, 'the heaviest mortality occurs in North Wales – where one might have surmised that the mountain air and other conditions would make for healthy living. ...' He went on to ask what could be responsible for the

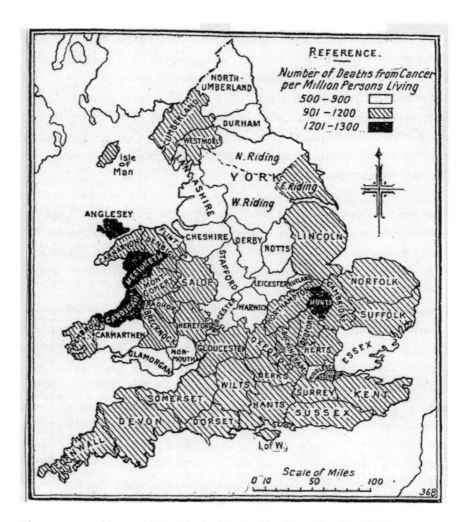

The cancer map of 1914, published in the 'blue book' and reproduced in *The Times*.

differences: ' … is it in the climate, soil, in water, in wind current, in situation, in diet that the explanation will be found?'

The county variations were due, of course, to Britain's pattern of industrialisation. The areas with the lowest rates of cancer were those where industrialisation and urbanisation were greatest, and where men and women tended to die younger because of accidents at work and illnesses associated with poverty and urban working-class life. The death rate from cancer was lower, simply because people died from other causes before cancers could develop. By contrast, in rural and suburban areas where the local inhabitants had longer life expectancies there were higher rates of cancer. Macmillan, the public health practitioner, was posing poignant questions that needed to be answered. He did not answer them himself and nor could he, but he was also making the point that there was little or no research going on that would lead to answers. He had no confidence in the priorities of much established cancer research.

In the last *Crusade* pamphlet, Macmillan returned to his attack on vivisection. Apart from the humane and moral objections to experiments on live animals, he also pursued the arguments of Bell, Stenson Hooker and other doctors that vivisection was not in any event a productive avenue for cancer research. It is not necessary here to examine these arguments in detail. But it is worth noting that among many doctors there was a wider concern about the direction of the Cancer Research Fund under Bashford[14] and his successor. The Fund's work was almost all based on cell research in the laboratory using specially bred mice. Some leading specialists wanted the focus to be shifted to the human subject and in particular to the patient in the clinic. This would be one reason for the emergence of the British Empire Cancer Campaign in 1923 as an alternative cancer research institution.

The *Crusade* pamphlets were complemented by the *Popular Cancer Crusade Lectures*, given with the aid of the magic lantern, an early projection device. A few of the topics covered were the prevention of cancer, health in the home, the impact of environment and habits and modern medical thought. These lectures were intended to raise awareness about cancer to the man in the street. They were made available to clubs, societies and institutions. The first public magic lantern lecture was given by Charles Forward at The Polytechnic in Regent Street (now the University of Westminster) on 13 November 1914, and many followed. Forward's theme was usually 'Cancer – its causes and prevention', and it doubtless followed his well-known approach to the subject. Later reports record that the lectures were particularly popular with co-operative women's guilds, and that interestingly, audiences were mainly of working-class people.

The Society also produced a quarterly publication of news and information for its members and supporters called *The Journal of Cancer*.

This was a serious production, with editions including articles about aspects of cancer prevention, book reviews, items of news about cancer treatments from home and overseas, and reports from cancer hospitals. Altogether the output of information from the Society was substantial. Macmillan would later say, with characteristic humility, that this work made just a humble contribution to fighting the menace of cancer. But he would also point out that the Imperial Cancer Research Fund and the cancer hospitals were doing little, if anything, to educate the public about this awful disease. It is true that some of the information about cancer put out by the Society was wrong, but that is easy to appreciate in hindsight. At the time, many authorities, medical and non-medical, were similarly wrong in the things they said. There were in those days very few certainties about cancer, apart from its growing toll of suffering.

There were two more things that the new Society needed to do to establish itself as a serious organisation of its day. It needed to adopt an emblem or badge of distinction, and it needed to agree a Society motto. At its last meeting in 1913, the executive decided that its emblem would be a drawing of the ancient statue of Apollo which once stood in the Cortile del Belvedere in the Vatican City.[15] Apollo was the Roman God of light and truth, and of medicine and healing. Its significance is clear enough. The Society wanted to throw the light of day on, and search for the truth about, cancer and its treatments. The Society's motto, to be printed around the drawing of Apollo, was to be the ancient proverb *nullum numen abest si sit prudentia*, meaning *where there is prudence, there will be divine protection*. In other words, knowledge and a prudent lifestyle would prevent cancer, and of course, prevention is better than cure.

The first of the twentieth-century's two world wars began in August 1914, just twenty months after the Society had met formally for the first time. The war would have a devastating impact on the Society's progress. The public mind turned, not surprisingly, to the cataclysmic events that were unfolding across the English Channel, and to the huge number of soldiers of the Empire killed or wounded in battle. Deaths from cancer, even if they were increasing, could not be compared with the appalling loss of young life that would touch every village and every urban street in the United Kingdom. The Society's messages about cancer just could

THE SECOND

ANNUAL REPORT

AND

YEAR BOOK

OF THE

SOCIETY FOR THE PREVENTION AND RELIEF OF CANCER.

For the Year ending December 31st,

1913.

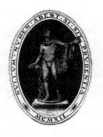

LONDON :
15 RANELAGH ROAD,
BELGRAVIA, S.W.

Annual Report and Yearbook for 1913 – the Apollo Belvedere is inset.

not penetrate the public mind. Moreover, the Society's leading figures were themselves busy with war work.[16] As a result, the four years of war were years of little activity for cancer prevention or relief. The Society continued to meet, but its income was cut to a trickle. The charity-giving public turned their generosity towards organisations that were supporting war relief. From the high in 1913 of £187, income fell to a low of just £36 in 1917 (about £2,200 today). The Society was not even able to distribute copies of its journal or its leaflets because it could not afford the cost of postage. The war hit the Society personally too when Lt Charles Deards, serving in the Royal Flying Corps, a member of the Society's council and its honorary solicitor, was killed in action over France.

The end of the First World War in November 1918 did not bring much greater fortune to the Society. Income did not rise appreciably, if at all, despite plans to raise funds through events as varied as concerts and boxing contests, the distribution of charity collecting boxes and sales of goods. A little grant aid came from the London County Council. However, no new members were recruited to the Society, and so through deaths and resignations the number of members actually fell. There was clearly a limit to the financial support that could come from Margaret Macmillan. With little income, there could be little cancer prevention and relief activity, and in 1922 the *Journal of Cancer* was abandoned. It is clear from the minutes of the Society's meetings that Macmillan himself was despairing about the Society's future. Indeed, the Society was close to collapse altogether, and it could well have disappeared along with thousands of other small charities that have come and gone without much notice. It was the Society's darkest hour.

There are several explanations for why the Society failed to grow in the immediate postwar years. First, the Society had no paid staff and had to rely entirely on the voluntary work of the two Macmillans, Forward, Mackenzie Bell and the others, most of whom also had business commitments and other interests. The Society had insufficient manpower to give it the critical mass it needed to make an impact. Second, the Society was caught in a trap that is familiar to many small charities. It is difficult to raise money without some evidence of charitable activity to show to potential donors, and it is impossible to undertake much charitable activity without money. These early years of the Society were long before government grants and lottery funds were available to kick-start worthy projects and sustain their basic costs. Third, the Society's role as a ginger group on the fringe of the medical world just did not have sufficient attraction to draw in supporters. The Society's trenchant views on vivisection and vegetarianism would have alienated many people, not least those from the medical world, but also from society as a whole for whom eating meat was regarded not just as normal, but as very healthy. It was, after all, the poor who could not afford to eat meat and it was the poor who suffered most from disease generally and who died young. Macmillan's charity therefore had too narrow an appeal, and doubtless many others thought it was too eccentric or too radical. Ironically, it would be the founding of another cancer charity – the British Empire Cancer Campaign – that would help the Society to set on a new course.

Notes & References

1. The Independent Order of Good Templars was a temperance organisation founded in the United States of America in 1854, and which had a strong following in Scotland.
2. From the Sidcot School website, 2005.
3. Interview with Joan Bebbington on 6 June 2005.
4. Quoted from 'Interview with the Founder', *Cancer Relief Bulletin*, Spring 1938.
5. Quoted from *The Book of Cancer*, published by NSCR, 1951.
6. Quoted from National Society for Cancer Relief report, 1931.
7. Although the first literature for the society was produced in 1912, and its first recorded meeting was held that year, it has always been assumed that preliminary work began in 1911. For this reason, 1911 has usually been regarded as the year of the society's foundation. The society's diamond jubilee was held in 1971.
8. See *Animal Rights* by Hilda Keen, published by Reakton Books, 1998.
9. See *The Cancer Blackout* by Nat Morris, published by Regent House, LA, 1977, and also correspondence between Murray and C.H. Mitchell re-printed in *The Journal of Cancer*, Vol. II, April 1920.

10. The first annual meeting also elected a smaller executive to deal with matters between meetings of the council. This structure lasted until the Society became a limited company in 1989.

11. For a full account of the trial before Lord Alverstone, CJ, see reports in *The Times*, 12, 13 and 14 June 1912.

12. *The Lancet*, 30 April 1864, p. 511; referred to in *The People's Health* by F.B. Smith, published by Croom Helm, 1979.

13. Under the Infectious Diseases (Notification) Act 1889, doctors were required to report to the local authority all cases of certain infectious diseases so that the authority could take action to prevent further infection.

14. Ernest Bashford, aged 41, resigned as director of the fund in 1914 because of ill health. He nevertheless served as a captain in the army for the duration of the Great War and died in 1923. Although not without his critics, he was one of the leading, if not the leading, cancer researcher of his time.

15. The statue is now in the Vatican's Pio–Clementino Museo.

16. Forward went to the war zone in Europe as a volunteer with Our Dumb Friends League, caring for injured horses. The League is now the Blue Cross.

3

A Welfare Charity

The creation of the British Empire Cancer Campaign brought cancer research to a higher level of activity, both in terms of scope and finance. A number of the leading doctors had become unhappy with the direction and progress of the Imperial Cancer Research Fund. These included John Lockhart–Mummery, a surgeon at St Mark's Hospital in London; Sir Thomas Horder, of the Royal Marsden Hospital, who believed in bringing together research from the clinic and the laboratory; the king's physician Lord Dawson of Penn; and Home Office pathologist Sir Bernard Spilsbury. They planned a new cancer charity, and one that would go beyond laboratory-based cell research. The British Red Cross agreed to launch an appeal for £1 million for this new cancer research charity, and other backers pledged substantial sums.

The new charity was launched in a letter to *The Times* on 30 May 1923. The letter pointed out that, despite all the advances that had been made in understanding cancer and in treating the disease, no progress at all had been made in identifying its causes. Such a statement must surely have received the fullest endorsement from Douglas Macmillan and his colleagues in the Society. The causes of cancer, the letter to *The Times* promised, would be an important area of study for the new charity. Its founders also promised a multi-disciplinary and inclusive approach to its research, unlike the Imperial Cancer Research Fund, which was exclusively medical.

With the British Empire Cancer Campaign gathering a swell of support, it was clear to Macmillan that it would be impossible for his society, already seriously compromised, to continue as a separate body with objectives that so clearly overlapped. A priority for the Society had, after all, always been to identify the causes of cancer and, through education and the spread of information, to help people protect themselves against the disease.

Consequently, on behalf of the Society, Macmillan wrote on 2 July 1923 to the chairman of the new charity, Lockhart-Mummery, describing the work of the Society from its beginnings and inviting any proposals that he might wish to make for its future. Some form of affiliation or even amalgamation must have been options in Macmillan's mind. Macmillan said on behalf of the Society that,

> We have no axe to grind, and desire only to see a determined and comprehensive campaign against 'the black scourge'.[1] My personal position in the matter is that this is 'spare time' work, carried out in the scanty leisure which follows a normally busy day elsewhere. In one sense therefore it would be a relief to me to know that the work to which we put our hands twelve years ago was being carried out with equal zeal, and far more adequately, by others.

On the other hand, Macmillan made it clear that the Society would want to be satisfied before it threw its lot in with the Campaign that the full range of its work would be carried forward. Macmillan's letter put this work in two parts:

> first, popular educational work, giving the common people the best possible advice in all matters relating to the prevention, diagnosis, treatment and relief of cancerous diseases; and second, practical relief work, such as the provision of hospital wards, beds, or cottage hospitals, and in necessitous cases of bandages, dressings, &c.

It is no surprise that Macmillan expressed in this letter his personal relief that a new organisation might take over the work of the Society. The Society's income in 1922 had been just £39. He must have understood that there was no possibility of the Society making any impact on cancer prevention or relief while its supporter base was so small and its resources so meagre.

A reply to Macmillan's letter, with a proposal for the future direction of the Society, came in a letter dated 26 November from the secretary of the new charity, Colonel Ernest Chapman. It read:

> ... the objects of your society are two-fold. Firstly, the prevention of Cancer by circulation of information on the subject, and secondly, the relief of Cancer patients by monetary or other assistance.
>
> ... we think the very best suggestion that could be made ... would be that you should cease from the first part ... and devote your whole energies to the second part, which I believe is not covered by any other charitable organisation. There are undoubtedly thousands of cases of Cancer where some organisation to enable them to have easy transport to the proper hospitals, either for operative treatment or X-ray, and their after care, especially in the cases where the patient has no hopes, or very small hopes, of recovery, would be an excellent charity, and would do an immense amount of good if support could be obtained.

This suggestion from the British Empire Cancer Campaign, despite the rather convoluted language of its secretary, clearly did not see the Society as having any mainstream role in cancer prevention or cancer information. It was rather to be sidelined into a provider of hospital transport, though there can be no doubt that this was an important gap in services at the time. However, the general idea of the Society concentrating its efforts on welfare was accepted, and the Society for the Prevention and Relief of Cancer evolved into the National Society for Cancer Relief.

The metamorphosis from a society primarily concerned with cancer prevention, to a society primarily dedicated to cancer relief took some months to complete. A new constitution had to be drafted and, to give the Society a greater degree of public scrutiny, it was decided to apply for registration with the Registrar of Friendly Societies. This was an unusual step for a welfare charity, but it probably arose from the Society's structure as a membership-based organisation as much as its new focus on relief. A good proportion of the Society's income had come from annual membership subscriptions, and if this were to be increased then increasing the size of the membership was an essential precondition. The oversight and regulation that came with Friendly Society status would add to the Society's credibility. The Society was finally registered as a benevolent society on 1 December 1924, and given the number 1665. The new constitution and rules, having lost the references to vivisection and diet, were adopted at the Annual General Meeting held that year. Interestingly, despite the decision to withdraw from preventative work, the new constitution still included as one of the objectives of the Society a sentence about preventing cancer. Perhaps Macmillan and his colleagues intended to leave their long-term options open. If the new British Empire Research Campaign did not come up with the goods, they could always go back to this work themselves. But meanwhile, Chapman was right; the relief of people suffering from cancer was a wholly neglected area of work, although helping the less wealthy with their travel costs to hospitals was just one small part of it.

Public welfare provision between the two world wars was still rudimentary and far from comprehensive or even adequate. The welfare state was still some years away. In 1908 the Liberal government of Herbert Henry Asquith had introduced old age pensions of 5s. per week (less than £20 today) for those over 70 years of age and without other financial means. This was sufficient, just, to keep old people out of the workhouse, but it was not anywhere near enough to maintain anyone with a basic standard of living, let alone someone coping with cancer. In 1911 the same government passed the National Insurance Act which, for the first time, provided compulsory sickness insurance through friendly societies for most working men and women. There was a sickness benefit rate of 10s. a week and disablement benefit of 5s. per week. Again, these rates were pretty miserly and unlikely to meet the needs of someone seriously ill. The sickness insurance scheme also included free medical treatment for the insured worker from a 'panel doctor', but this did not extend to the insured worker's family. People needing welfare or medical care, and who fell through the net of the Liberal reforms, unless they had other means of support, would still have to rely on the workhouse or the outdoor relief of the Poor Law, suffering all the shame and indignity that came with it. For many, this was to be avoided for as long as earthly possible. One doctor at the Middlesex Hospital recorded the case of a husband and father,

> seen at the cancer outpatients department in an almost dying condition from an ulcerated cancer of the throat. The reason he assigned for not seeking earlier advice was that he was afraid of losing his job and bringing his family to want. This instance of heroic capacity for 'sticking it' to the end is not an isolated, nor even a very rare one.[2]

This was an example of extraordinary human fortitude but, surely, one of very many. The only other hope for people doubly inflicted by cancer and poor circumstances was charity.

The challenge to the Society to make an impact on the welfare of people with cancer, and particularly poor people, was a mighty and daunting one, but also one that was hugely worthwhile. Disappointingly, a programme of cancer relief was slow to develop. Some very limited relief work was reported during the years of the Great War, but no details have survived. The first recorded recipient of help from the Society was Mr Horace Craske, a patient at the West Beckton Infirmary in Norfolk with cancer in the neck. A payment of 10 guineas (i.e. £10.50) was made to meet medical fees, and the Society arranged for him to be moved to a hospital in Norwich for surgery. This was in June 1925. Craske, who was thought to have been cured, wrote to the Society with his appreciation for the help that he had received, and the council was so pleased to hear about this that it reported the story to the ultra-patriotic *John Bull* magazine.

The Society's council also agreed that the executive and the secretary should have delegated authority to make grants in cases of emergency. Nevertheless, expenditure on relief and welfare remained very modest and no more than a handful of patients were helped in the following several years. Of these few, two were London cases reported in 1928. The first was a 70-year-old woman with cancer of the breast. The Society's voluntary worker reported that:

From April until June I visited her. … Her only daughter had just passed away. Her husband was very sickly, and unfortunately was knocked down and died some weeks later from the effects. They had just enough to pay the rent of two rooms and procure the bare necessities of life. The old lady craved for fresh eggs and fruit, which I took. She was so grateful and her one trouble was that she might be taking the things from someone not so well off as herself. She was ultimately removed to the Infirmary, where she died last December.

The second case was of a 60-year-old widow with intestinal cancer, who lived with a daughter and four grandchildren, all in appalling poverty. Again, the voluntary worker reported:

She was practically starving. I made arrangements for such things as fish, milk puddings etc. to be supplied to her, cooked. She called for it every day, and then we tried to get it to her. I also supplied her with a pound of cotton wool every week. She had to be taken to the Infirmary. While she was there I sent her tea, fresh butter, and things she could not afford to buy herself. She was very grateful for the help; it was, I think, the one bright spot in her very sordid existence, and she could hardly believe it.

In 1928 the Society spent just £1 17s. 2d. on patient welfare; a ridiculously small amount of money. It really was a teaspoonful of help in an ocean of need. And even this ocean of need must have grown markedly with the financial collapse of 1929 and the economic depression that followed. Unemployment rose to a level not seen for fifty years, state welfare benefits were reduced, and most incomes were squeezed during what came to be known as the 'hungry thirties'. For the jobless and the poor these were years of hardship, the likes of which have not been seen since.

The reason for the Society's relief work remaining so modest was that the Society's income continued to bump along the bottom. Many initiatives to raise money were pursued with variable success, but none were on a scale large enough to drive up income to a level that would allow the Society to have a meaningful impact on the problem. Several applications were made to the BBC for the Society to be the subject of a radio appeal, but without immediate results. There were efforts to boost membership and to encourage those making wills to leave a gift to the Society. Sales of goods and benefit performances were taken up when the opportunities arose. Charles Forward continued with his lecture programme, but made a charge of 10s. 6d. for each one. At the end of 1930 the Society had only seventy members and an income for the year of less than £42. It was not without a great deal of realism that George B. Ireland of Totnes in Devon, one of the original subscribers to the Society, and doubtless exasperated after eighteen years of extremely modest achievement, wrote to the Annual General Meeting held in that year calling for the Society to be wound up.

The response of the Society was a milestone in its history. It decided, at last, to appoint a full-time and paid officer to take responsibility for raising funds. Some sixty people replied to a newspaper advertisement for the post described as assistant secretary and, from a shortlist of four, Reginald Gollop was appointed at a meeting held on 6 November 1930. Gollop was a man of strong religious faith and so most likely got on well with Macmillan. More importantly, he had previous experience of charity fund-raising as a paid collector with the Friends of the Poor.[3]

Gollop's appointment radically changed the fortunes of the Society. He would remain with the Society, later taking on the role of secretary when Macmillan became chairman, until his death from cancer in January 1952.[4] Gollop set about raising income through house to house collections, and he began to build a national organisation for the Society with the appointment of local collectors in the larger towns of England. He also actively sought new members. By the end of 1931, his first year, income had risen to £3,295 (about £137,000 today), and the Society had 200 members. Five years later, income was up to £10,206 and there were 600 members. By the outbreak of the Second World War, income had doubled again to £20,720. This was growth on a scale never before experienced by the Society. Gollop and his expanding team of organisers and collectors almost certainly saved the Society from just fading away.

The financial growth of the Society allowed it to expand its welfare work into a more worthwhile service across several parts of the UK. Two hundred and fifty-six patients were given assistance of one sort or another in 1935, costing the Society £1,672. Five hundred and forty-two people were helped in 1939, at a cost of £9,131. In reality, the Society was still doing little more than putting a small dent into a very large surface of need, but it was work of extraordinary comfort for those patients who were able to benefit. One early case history drew a parallel to the patient who attended the outpatient clinic of the Middlesex Hospital those few years before. According to the Society's 1931 report the patient was a

> comparatively young widow who had worked as a temporary clerk in Government offices, and became aware, two years ago, that cancer was in her breast. She obtained radium and other treatment at the hospitals, but the growth continued to spread. Her service did not qualify her for a pension, and her son was earning but a trifle. 'I have tried unsuccessfully for some kind of light employment,' she wrote, 'as it is my wish to be self-supporting as long as possible. ... I wonder if you could possibly put me in touch with anyone who could utilise my services for a few hours daily?' Enquiries showed however, that she was quite unfit to do outside work, her few domestic duties and her own dressings being sufficiently exhausting. She dreaded being sent into a hospital as she could not then keep a home together for her boy. The home was found to consist of two little rooms in the City of London, in a small building inhabited by twenty-six families! A clean spot in dirty surroundings. A weekly pension was awarded her by the Society, but the malady steadily worsened, and in a couple of months the plucky struggle was ended. We had her own assurance that a big load was lifted from this sufferer's mind by the little aid we were able to give, and we could only regret that it had not been sought sooner.

For the most part, support for patients came in the form of a weekly pension or allowance of between 2s. 6d. and £1 (between about £6 and £42 today) which was paid until the patient died. Quite often, patients would be in receipt of this pension for many months or even years. Grants were also given for medicines and dressings, bedding and clothing, nursing care and convalescence, travel costs, artificial limbs, and most importantly in the days before domestic central heating, hot water bottles. The annual reports of the Society list case after case of patients whom the Society had been able to help. Case histories were also used in fund-raising and other promotional literature. Each case history was compiled by one of the Society's workers. Each tells its own story of sadness and distress, with the hope that the Society had been able to alleviate the suffering in some little way.

Below are the stories of just a few patients who were helped and supported by the Society in these years. Some stories are distressing to read even after nearly eighty years. They are included only to give an accurate reflection of the appalling suffering that could accompany cancer and that was sadly not uncommon just two or three generations ago.

Mr H: *this man's nose is being eaten away – a ghastly sight*

Mrs B: *a refined woman who had suffered bankruptcy and years of ill-health. Her pains so acute that she frequently screamed and wept. Her daughter used £10 worth of dressings every week. The foul smell was really fearful …*

Poor woman: *(46), with 3 children, deserted by husband. Needed nourishing foods and general help.*

Little girl: *(9) one of twelve children. Mother had only 30/- per week to feed and clothe herself, husband and seven children; two of whom had no shirts to wear. Child's disease aggravated by severe chest cold caused by sleeping in kitchen bed facing door in a bleak district. … Parents refused to let her be nursed at Infirmary.*

Boy: *(6), condition hopeless. Parents asked to visit him in hospital daily but could not afford fares.*

Mrs P: *I shall never forget this patient; a woman who had been very good looking. … A terrible case to visit; a relief nurse had to give it up. Cancer was spreading over her face, and the flies irritated her tremendously. She had no dressing on her face, her nose was crumbling away and she could only take liquids through a tube.*

Lonely widow: *(76), trying desperately to keep free of debt, needs fuel and foods.*

Poor blind woman: *(53), husband incapacitated and unemployed. Income inadequate to meet needs.*

Small girl: *(7), has been in hospital for over a year. Parents had large family to provide for and needed help with fares.*

Poor woman: *husband a T.B. patient, only daughter an epileptic. Needed special foods.*

Woman: (56), with no income (husband committed suicide leaving debts), had melanotic sarcoma of foot necessitating amputation of right leg, and required artificial limb. Society contributed £10 towards cost.

Old couple: living in one room, and both afflicted with malignant growths. Wife should have operation but unable to leave husband. Both needing proper nourishment.

Man: (56), with cancer of the lung, following damage by shrapnel in 1914–18 war. Lives with bed-ridden sister of 75: no one to look after him. Unfit for work and outlook hopeless.

The stories also express, quite movingly, how many of the people that the Society was able to help were quite overcome with gratitude. **Mr P**, a man with cancer of the tongue, wrote to the Society's worker to say,

> I cannot put into words how grateful I am to you for your kindness to me. I did not think there were people like you in this world of ours, for your kind assistance to me, a stranger, for practically no asking. ... No doubt you are aware nobody wants your company when you have got a dreaded disease like I have got.

Mr H: *A family of four, father suffering from Cancer of the Lung, the wife suffering from ill-health, totally blind in one eye, a little daughter almost blind in both eyes, and a little son who is almost blind and an imbecile. The total income of this family is 15/9 per week, and out of it they have to pay 10/- rent. The father, mother and little daughter are sleeping in one bed.*

> *Before the Society heard of this case, these poor things were almost destitute, neighbours were supplying them with pieces of bread, little bits of butter etc. The wife on being informed that the Society had decided to allow the husband a weekly pension was almost too crushed to express her gratitude.*

Perhaps the most perverse and fatalistic of cases was that of two brothers, pioneers of X-ray machine technology, who had been contracted to maintain the X-ray equipment at a London hospital. A reporter of the *Daily Express* wrote in 1933 that they were,

> paying a heavy price for their devotion to science in the early days when little was known of the destructive powers of the rays that now heal.

George started making X-ray tubes thirty-five years ago. One of Harley Street's most eminent radiologists told me that these two men had played a conspicuous part in the advancement of this work in its early stages. They were often called in by specialists when anything went wrong with the X-ray apparatus. That service was always given voluntarily.

The business which the two brothers carried on for years in connection with X-ray work has had to be closed down. Both are practically penniless; there is no fund, apparently, they can call on to aid them in their troubles.

George, the elder, is trying gamely to re-start life afresh. ... He is heavily handicapped. One of his eyes has been burned out; he has had three internal haemorrhages.

Bert, the other brother, is lying in the hospital. He has lost three fingers and another is doomed. He has had a series of glandular operations.

Both men were suffering from cancers brought about by excessive exposure to radiation, at a time when the carcinogenic nature of radiation was not understood. Having no other means of support these men, who had been in the frontline of cancer treatment, were awarded by the Society pensions for life.

The Society's programme of welfare, which became known in shorthand as 'patient grants', needed a professional structure to support it, and it needed too, the cooperation of local hospitals and welfare services. At the beginning, visits to all patients were carried out by volunteers, but in 1932, two full-time paid visitors were appointed to cover two key centres of Society activity: Mrs Lilian Castle was appointed to cover London; and Mrs Ruth Hurn was appointed to work in York. To help Mrs Hurn travel around her area, she was given use of a Society bicycle – the modest forerunner of the company car. Two years later, part-time paid visitors were appointed to work in the areas of Hastings, Windsor and Ipswich. Volunteers, who despite this status still held official appointments, covered Bolton, Cardiff and Swansea. Local clergymen were also recruited to help the Society in its work. By the outbreak of the Second World War, the Society's network of visitors covered many, though by no means all, parts of England, Scotland and Wales.

It was hard work for the visitors. Mrs Castle reported in 1938 that she had forty-three patients on her books. Apart from home visits, she had needed to visit forty different hospitals, including all the major London institutions, make many calls on clergy and other almoners, doctors and district nurses, and collect and distribute gifts of clothing, linen and even furniture. In the same year, Mrs Hurn had made 2,473 visits to her patients. Mrs Hurn built strong links with the York City Health Department and was able to get the use of facilities in the York Dispensary and of the city ambulance to transport her patients to the radium centre at Leeds where they could receive radiotherapy treatment. In many ways, the Society's visitors of the 1930s were the Macmillan nurses of their time. They provided practical help and assistance to patients and their families and also emotional support. A visitor in the south of England said of her patients,

> The relief these poor souls enjoy in many ways is really wonderful. Most of them were poorly clad, but we have been able to supply outdoor clothes as well as bed-clothes. The regular visiting has helped to improve the home conditions, too. ... Then with extra white lint and cotton wool they are able to change the dressings oftener and are more comfortable. I always put a new case in touch with a Minister, if they haven't one already, and a visit is regularly paid by him.

The limited manpower of the Society, paid and voluntary, inevitably restricted the geographical scope of its welfare work. It is true that many hospitals in major towns (including even the British Hospital in Paris) would, on payment by the Society, provide continuing supplies of dressings and appliances and extra supplies of foods to poor patients discharged home. At the same time, the Society would work in collaboration with other charities, such as The Salvation Army and the British Legion, and with local guilds. But the Society's reach remained patchy. In 1938, for example, while twenty-two patients living in Suffolk received support, for Lincolnshire the figure was only three. In Macmillan's ancestral Scotland, just nine patients received some help from the Society. No patients at all were helped in Staffordshire and Nottinghamshire, while ninety-seven from Lancashire received support

Report on the

CANCER RELIEF

Work of the N.S.C.R. in 1932.

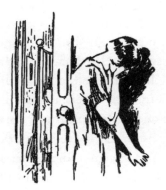

HELP

has been freely given to a greatly increased number of poor sufferers in 1932.

HELP

is constantly needed to enable us to maintain and extend our services to necessitous victims of disease and poverty.

Report of the Society, 1932.

and 152 from Yorkshire. The Society had a long way to go before it could be true to its description of 'national'.

With patient welfare becoming the central focus of the Society's activities, the Society's emblem of Apollo and its motto about the wisdom of prevention were no longer appropriate. They were dropped in 1924. In 1931 a new emblem appeared, consisting of a drawing of a woman, deeply distressed, standing just outside the door of an occupied bedroom. This was a powerful image, reflecting the anguish, pain and despair that accompanied cancer, both for the patient and for the family. From this time, the Society was more often called, in shorthand, *Cancer Relief*, and this name would stick until the 1990s.

Perhaps one last patient is worth mentioning. In 1927 Macmillan and Charles Forward told the story of a 35-year-old woman with breast cancer. She was the wife of a labourer earning just £2 per week; they had two children and lived in great poverty. She had discharged herself early from the Infirmary following surgery. Her doctor told the Society that in order to build up her strength she needed, among other things, meat extracts. Despite the Society's roots in vegetarianism, it provided the needy patient with the meat extracts. Macmillan and Forward may have had their opinions about the consumption of meat, but the Society had moved on from its early days as a campaigner for vegetarianism.

Douglas Macmillan was always closely and personally involved with the welfare work of the Society. He was chairman of the committee which awarded the grants and annuities and he had the authority to take decisions between formal committee meetings. He took this responsibility very seriously, taking every opportunity to acquaint himself with the details of the cases. He was also one of the Society's voluntary workers who often visited patients in their homes. This gave him an acute knowledge of the nursing and welfare needs of patients and of their families, and he used this knowledge as the basis for much of his campaigning work. One of his helpers from this time recalled some fifty years later,

> He used to visit a cancer patient in her home and often he would take me with him. We walked the two miles as he did not have a car, spend about one hour sitting at her bedside and then the two miles home. I

realise now what a privilege it was to have known such a gentle and unassuming man. Much of our conversation then was what he hoped for in the years ahead. ...[5]

Notes & References

1. The 'black scourge' was a common expression to describe cancer. The 'white scourge', or the 'white death', were expressions to describe tuberculosis.
2. From *Cancer Research at the Middlesex Hospital 1900–1924 Retrospect & Prospect*, edited by W. Sampson Handley, published 1924 by Middlesex Hospital Press.
3. The League of the Friends of the Poor was established in 1905 by the Church Army with a focus on self-help and support from better off members of society. It evolved into the charity of today called Friends of the Elderly.
4. When Gollop died, Macmillan wrote of his friendly and kindly manner, and said that the work he most enjoyed was patient welfare.
5. Jessie Squibb writing on 18 August 1984 in a letter to the secretary of the Society.

4

'I Want to See ...'

The financial welfare of patients with cancer may have become the focus of the Society's charitable work, but it did not wholly absorb the mind of Douglas Macmillan. His vision, and those of his colleagues, had always been much wider. From the beginning, Macmillan was interested in the medical and nursing treatment and care of patients, and since the publication of the 'blue book' he had campaigned for more and better cancer care facilities and services. However, between the world wars there was no comprehensive state health service in Britain. The Ministry of Health had been created in 1919, though not to universal approval, by drawing together the health care responsibilities of several other Whitehall departments. This made the coordination of government health activities, at least, more straightforward. Nevertheless, hospital and nursing services were still provided, quite independently of each other, by a range of local authority, private and charitable institutions. There was little or no planning of health services, and their financial support was complex and, for many, woefully inadequate. It is true that successive ministers of health, including the future prime minister

Neville Chamberlain, had argued for a greater coordination at local level of the providers of health services, and particularly hospital services, but little in practice was achieved before 1939.

At the top of the league for good cancer treatment and care were the few specialist cancer hospitals and specialist cancer wards of voluntary hospitals. But these were still very few in number. These were followed by the big voluntary general hospitals that had been established in many major cities during the eighteenth and nineteenth centuries, and sometimes even earlier. Many of these hospitals were also teaching establishments linked to the universities and they attracted the best medical and surgical practitioners. Young doctors passing out from these great hospitals often became the resident physicians and surgeons at the smaller voluntary hospitals.

All of the voluntary hospitals were essentially charitable and they often provided care freely to the poor and on a scale of fees according to a patient's means. They were funded by a mixture of endowments, donations and subscriptions. It was an interesting facet of the voluntary hospitals that the very best of them were quite often situated in, or near to, the areas of greatest poverty. Being poor did not necessarily mean that a patient would get the poorest medical care. The voluntary hospitals were at liberty to provide for the care of patients and for the treatments of diseases as were set out in their foundation deeds, or as their governing bodies might decide. However, it was common for the voluntary hospitals to concentrate on providing acute medical care. Patients needing long-term care would commonly fall outside of their admissions policy and be forced to go elsewhere. Mostly, these patients would go to the public hospitals operated by local authorities, or at worst in terms of quality, to the old Poor Law infirmaries.

The local authority or municipal hospitals had originally been set up under various public health acts to provide a quite specific range of care and treatments, in particular for mental health, maternity, infectious diseases and tuberculosis. Increasingly, they came to offer more wide-ranging medical and nursing care, including care for patients with cancer, but it was likely to be palliative and not curative treatment. Although most of the municipal hospitals employed resident surgeons, few of them were likely to be very experienced at excising cancers. The Poor Law infirmaries were originally provided as an adjunct to the workhouse, often caring for the old and disabled and the long-term chronic sick, and for those long beyond the hope of curative medicine or surgery. The standard of care was usually very low.

By the Local Government Act of 1929, the local authorities took over the Poor Law infirmaries and incorporated them into their own hospital services. This at least removed the stigma of poverty and destitution from those who had to enter them. The Act also allowed local authorities to expand their range of hospital services, but this part of the legislation was permissive only and a limited number of councils took advantage of its provisions. As a result, the distribution of the municipal hospitals was as irregular as that of the voluntary ones. Moreover, with local authorities giving preference of admission to their own residents, some people living almost on the doorstep of one municipal hospital, but just the other side of its local government boundary, might have to travel miles to another hospital that served the local authority in which they lived. The result was that hospital care and treatment for people with cancer – inpatients and outpatients – varied greatly from one part of the country to another. A cancer patient living close to the Middlesex Hospital in London, or the cancer hospital in Glasgow would, in all probability, receive the best treatment that medical science at the time had available, irrespective of his ability to pay. But cancer treatment and care in the municipal hospitals, and particularly in the old Poor Law establishments, could be very basic indeed.[1]

The chronic lack of national planning and coordination of health services was well demonstrated by the haphazard and random supply of radium, the radioactive element discovered by the Curies. Radium had become a mainstream treatment of cancer and it was commonly used, though with little evidence base and some danger to patients and staff, as an alternative to surgery. The element was derived, in the tiniest of quantities, from the mineral pitchblende. It was extremely expensive and in very short supply. One hospital official appealed to the Society for help: 'We have several urgent cases for Radium in this Hospital. ... It always means a long and hard struggle to get the money to procure it, and there are cases for which there should be no delay.'

The Society appreciated that there were doubtless many hospitals in the same predicament and it joined the campaign to support a central radium distribution agency. In response to this problem, the government set up in 1929, by charter, the National Radium Trust & Radium Commission. The commission augmented the supply of radium (its first purchase was of 13 grams of the substance) and concentrated radium supply in seventeen cancer treatment centres. This was the first attempt ever made to bring a rational approach to cancer treatment across Britain. It did though bring its own problems. Patients would have to travel to a radium centre to receive treatment, and this was prohibitive for the many people who were poor. The Society's own funds were nowhere near sufficient to provide a national hospital transport service. The Duke of York, later King George VI, as Patron of the British Empire Cancer Campaign, urged an appeal for funds to help poor patients with their travel expenses to the treatment centres. It was estimated that only 20 per cent of patients with cancers that were treatable with radium actually received this life prolonging therapy.

The same disparities existed in district nursing. In 1859 William Rathbone, a wealthy merchant in Liverpool, employed a nurse to work with the sick and poor of the city in their own homes, and he first used the term district nurse.[2] Other early schemes to care for the sick in their own homes were set up by charitable and religious bodies. One example was the London Bible and Domestic Female Mission founded by Mrs Ellen Ranyard. Her Bible nurses were the first trained district nurses in London and by the turn of the century they were visiting 10,000 patients a year.[3] Similar schemes were established in many towns across Britain, some giving emphasis to home nursing, but others concentrating more on preventative work. The Queen Victoria Institute for Nursing the Poor was founded in 1889 to provide training for this new breed of nurse, later called Queen's nurses. For state sponsored district nursing, however, the priorities tended to be the same as those of the public hospitals, such as public health and maternity, so only very limited services were available for cancer patients. The health insurance introduced by the 1911 National Insurance Act could be used for nursing at home, but only for the care of the insured worker and not his family. With the additional economic and financial strictures of the inter-war years, both the availability and the quality of nursing care at home were variable to say the least.

Against this background in 1930 the Society, doubtless inspired by
Macmillan, re-opened its campaign for better cancer treatment and
care services. The Society took the statistics from the General Registry
of England and Wales to show that in the twenty years between 1909
and 1929, cancer deaths in England and Wales had increased again, this
time by 67 per cent. This was sure proof of Macmillan's much-repeated
argument that the figures were not just the result of better diagnosis,
since the range of diagnostic tools had not changed significantly
during the period. And in its report for the year 1931 the society asked
rhetorically:

> What is the position today ... ? In 1930 alone, there died from cancer in
> England and Wales no fewer than 57,833 persons, *or three times the total
> number of deaths occurring on both sides in the whole course of the Boer
> War* [1899–1902] ...

Including cancer deaths in Scotland, nearly 70,000 had died from the
disease. The discourse continued with evidence to show that Macmillan's
prophesy of 1913, that cancer would overtake tuberculosis as a cause of
mortality, had not only been correct – it had happened in 1919 – but that
now, 'the death-rate from cancer is *almost double that of consumption*'.

On top of this, for the first time, there was an estimate of the
number of people at any one time who would have cancer. The Society
concluded that '*there must be something like half-a-million victims
of the malady in our midst today*'. It is not clear how this figure was
calculated, but it was supposed to include people with the disease in its
earliest stages and prior to diagnosis. The number may well have been
an exaggeration given the likely prognosis of the disease at that time (six
years later the Ministry of Health estimated that 100,000 people were
living with the disease but this figure was of cases diagnosed). However,
even allowing for some licence, the magnitude of the figure – equivalent
to the population of Leeds, or of Bristol and Bath together – must have
had a considerable impact on the reader.

Since the advances in public health in the latter part of the nineteenth
century, local authorities had been encouraged to make particular
provision for the treatment of patients with tuberculosis. As a result

beds in public hospitals were allocated for TB cases and, in addition, a number of voluntary bodies built TB sanitaria in out-of-town places with clean and salubrious air. The Society made the obvious contrast between the facilities available for TB patients and those for cancer patients. Macmillan calculated that there were 24,000 hospital beds set aside for patients with tuberculosis. But, adding together all of the beds available in the specialist cancer hospitals and wards, there were only 600 of them. The Society declared that, 'For every 100 patients dying of consumption, there are over 80 beds. *For every 100 patients dying of Cancer, there is barely 1 bed.*'

Of course, many people with cancer would be cared for in the general medical and surgical wards of public and voluntary hospitals, although as we have seen, the supply and distribution of these facilities was inadequate and haphazard. But the Society was very effectively making the point that despite the ever-growing scale of the cancer problem, it was not being tackled directly or specifically, or with sufficient urgency. In 1932 the Society reported that of ninety patients with cancer applying for admission to the Royal Edinburgh Hospital for Incurables, only sixty-four could be accommodated. Of the others, sixteen had died before a bed became available, and five were too ill to be moved. There is no reason to believe that these circumstances in Edinburgh were any different to most other parts of Britain. Indeed, they may well have been rather better.

The Society recognised, and it urged others to recognise, that the need for specific cancer services would most likely be long term, and that an all-embracing cure was not an immediate or even a foreseeable prospect. Looking at the progress of cancer research, the Society still held Macmillan's scepticism about its methods and the likelihood of success. The Society's report for 1931 opined:

> Possibly as much is being attempted in this country, and throughout the world, as can reasonably be expected in the way of experimental work, involving, as it does, the compulsory assistance of many thousands of animals. While few would grudge the heaviest financial sacrifices necessary to establish a cure, it has to be admitted that a cure is not yet, and may not even be near. Surgery has performed miracles, while radium

Report, 1931.

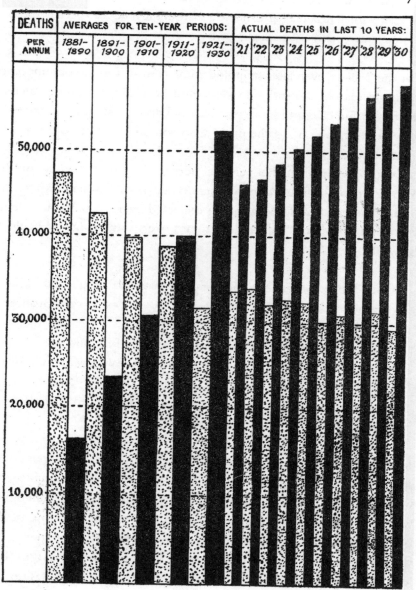

The " dotted " pillars represent the annual death-rates from CONSUMPTION, and the black pillars the corresponding rates from CANCER. The first part of the diagram shows the remarkable manner in which the relative deadliness of the two diseases has been reversed in the last 40 years.

Campaigning for more hospital places for cancer patients, 1930.

is still on trial. There are some who hold that much more might have been learned regarding causation if a share of the funds had been devoted to intensive statistical and field work.

For the Society, even after stripping away its suspicion of contemporary cancer research, the only answer could be more resources put into treatment and care, and more particularly into care. If cure was indeed a long way off, the care of the many who could not be cured became an urgent need.

Douglas Macmillan, in a personal note in the 1931 report, set out his own vision for the future of cancer care. Based on his firsthand experience of the needs of people with cancer collected over the previous twenty years, and of patients 'appalling in their poverty, suffering and neglect', he wrote:

> I want ... to see a chain of 'homes' for cancer patients throughout the land, where attention will be provided freely or at low cost, as circumstances dictate.
> I want the poorest people to be provided with the latest and best advice both for avoiding cancer and for recognising and dealing with it when it exists.
> I want to see panels of voluntary nurses, who can be detailed off to attend to necessitous patients in their own homes.

This was an agenda for a radical and comprehensive improvement of cancer services, including, in particular, palliative care (although the term was not used at the time). The goals were ambitious and challenging, written as they were some fifteen years before the founding of the National Health Service, and in the very year that public expenditure was cut as the country sank deeper into economic depression. But Macmillan had always been a campaigner and in his three visions he set out challenges to the Society, and more widely to all who had responsibility for cancer services. Many would come later to similar conclusions, some inspired by Macmillan, and some not. But Douglas Macmillan's place among the pioneers of improved cancer and palliative care cannot be in dispute.

The provision of more inpatient facilities for cancer patients had always been an objective for the Society. As early as 1916 there had been discussions about the Society opening its own cancer hospital or nursing home, but the financial doldrums of the wartime years, and after, made the idea quite beyond hope. Further thought was given to the possibility in 1931, as the Society's income began to look much healthier. The idea had by then focused on the establishment being, more realistically, a nursing home rather than a hospital. It followed Macmillan's vision of 'homes for cancer patients' and a search for a suitable home began.

Properties were inspected at Hastings and St Leonards-on-Sea in East Sussex, where the Society had many subscribers, but the Society concluded that it would be better to search in the London area so that Douglas Macmillan could be close by to give the home some operational oversight. By this time, the Macmillans had moved to Sidcup, then just outside London in Kent (it is now a part of the London Borough of Bexley), and so the search moved to this area. In due course, in 1932, a property known as Park House in a small side street called The Park in Sidcup came onto the market. It no longer stands, but characteristic of the area are large, detached Victorian villas. Following a satisfactory building survey it was decided to acquire the property and a price of £1,250 was agreed. The Society then applied to Chislehurst Urban District Council for consent to use the property as a nursing home for patients with cancer.

The Society did not expect what followed. Some twenty-two residents of The Park and the adjacent Chislehurst Road presented a petition to the council protesting against the Society's proposals, primarily on the grounds that 'the rateable value of the neighbouring properties will be depreciated', and secondly because the property was unsuitable for such a use.[4] The local Conservative Member of Parliament, Walden Smithers, joined the campaign on the side of the residents. The Society responded by assuring the council that it would protect the amenity of the area. The council, doubtless not wishing to offend local residents, refused its consent.

There was an appeal to the Minister of Health and Local Government and an inspector held a public inquiry in July. Despite a case strongly argued by the Society's solicitor, the minister dismissed the appeal. The

Society's first attempt to operate a nursing home did not get off the ground. It must have been a great disappointment. But it may well have been a good thing. It is not at all certain that the Society had the skills and knowledge to manage such an establishment, and moreover the Society was becoming acutely aware of the financial commitments involved in maintaining and operating nursing homes. Some twenty years would pass before the Society would finally realise the ambition of acquiring and managing a nursing home. It may be a reflection on the fear and ignorance of cancer at the time that the presence of a small nursing home for cancer patients could depress local property values – putting such an establishment in much the same category as a bail hostel or travellers caravan site today. It certainly demonstrates that there is nothing recent about the public's 'not in my back yard' approach to health and social problems and their solutions.[5]

The Society did not withdraw from nursing home care altogether. An alternative help to patients was convalescence, a health service commonly available at the time but almost unheard of today. From 1938 the Society began to pay for patients to spend time convalescing from illness or treatment in one of several convalescent homes around the south coast. The Society even paid a retainer for the sole use by its patients of a three-bed female ward in a convalescent home on the Kent coast, until it was later requisitioned for war use.

Financial help towards convalescence or holidays became a regular part of the Society's patient welfare programme. Where the Society had a good relationship with the local authority, the city or county ambulance was offered at no cost to transport the patient to the convalescent home. In other cases, the Society had to pay. For many patients with cancer, sick or recovering, the opportunity to spend a week away at the English seaside was a rare opportunity and a great boost to health and morale. As late as 1986, the Society was to report that it had enabled,

> One man ... to go for the very first time in his life to the seaside. He had never even seen the sea before and nor had he ever stayed in a hotel. On his return he was so much stronger physically and had also taken huge mental leaps and bounds.

The steady growth of the cancer problem – it had become the second cause of death after heart disease – doubtless coupled with the agitation of the Society and many others for better and more comprehensive cancer services, did have an impact on the government. The outcome was the Cancer Act of 1939, a piece of legislation aimed specifically at improving access to cancer treatment and reducing the death toll of the disease. The Cancer Bill was introduced into parliament by the Minister of Health, Walter Elliot[6], in December 1938. Elliot had studied medicine and science at Glasgow University and in his inaugural review of his job he referred specifically to the 70,000 people who died each year from cancer and to what a challenge this was. Elliot reiterated that the death rate from the disease had increased from 835 per million living in 1901, to 1,624 per million living in 1937, and he accepted that the statistics could not be explained just by better diagnosis. He also drew attention to the death toll of those between the ages of 15 and 65, nearly one-fifth of which was caused by cancer, and when 'working or business capacity was at its fullest and when women and heads of families were most necessary to their children'.

Elliot was saying that fighting cancer was an economic as well as a humanitarian imperative. The purpose of the legislation was to improve the diagnosis and treatment of the disease by increasing the number of hospital cancer facilities. In Elliot's view, only London was adequately served. Elsewhere, long waiting times for diagnostic and treatment services meant that patients were seen when their cancer was no longer curable. The Ministry estimated that between 300 and 350 new centres would have to be established and staffed. It was an ambitious endeavour.

The new Act put the responsibility on local authorities to provide, either directly or with the voluntary hospitals, sufficient facilities for the diagnosis and treatment of cancer for people in their local areas. The Act also required local authorities to pay for the travel costs of patients attending the facilities for treatment, thereby removing one of the big hurdles that prevented access to treatment. Within twelve months of the Act attaining the Royal Assent on 29 March 1939, local authorities were required to submit their plans to the Minister of Health for approval. This was indeed a notable piece of legislation,

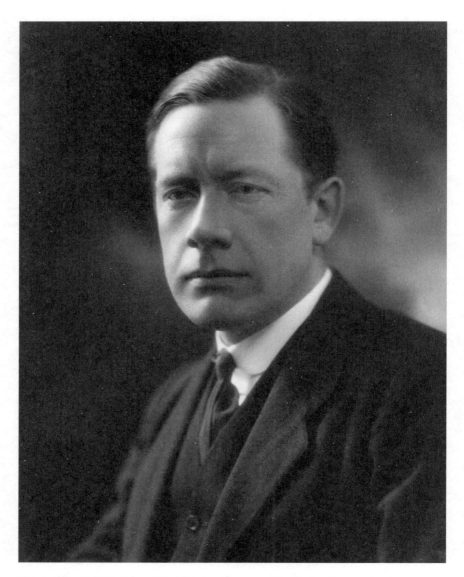

Walter Elliot MP, Minister of Health, who was responsible for the first cancer plan. (National Portrait Gallery)

at last making public authorities plan cancer diagnosis and treatment services. It pushed cancer services higher up the list of priorities, giving it the same importance as the control of tuberculosis and infectious diseases. The Act pledged central government funds phased over five years to help finance the new services, so local authorities could not plead a lack of cash as an excuse not to implement the legislation. The fate of the Act, however, lay not in the town halls of Great Britain, but in the Chancellery of Berlin. The outbreak of the Second World War, less than six months after the Act became law, meant that the priorities of central and local government changed overnight, and implementation of the Act became very difficult. Nevertheless, some progress was made in several areas, and the main purposes of the Act ultimately became, postwar, the responsibility of the National Health Service.

The Cancer Act represented an important recognition by the government of the scale of the cancer problem. It also recognised that treatments could be much more effective if patients began them at very early stages of the disease, and so it was essential that patients went for diagnosis and treatment as soon as any symptoms became noticeable. Walter Elliot was keen to conquer the 'bogy of incurability' and the dread of the disease that prevented people from seeking early medical advice. But he did understand that the biggest killers were cancers of the stomach and the intestines, which all too often did not give a patient any noticeable symptoms until it was too late. So, while the provisions of the Act were very welcome, they were far from comprehensive because they did not make any provision for the care of patients who were beyond curative treatments. In particular, the Act made no provision for the nursing care of patients at home, even though that was where many patients with terminal cancer were likely to be cared for by family members. The Society rightly observed that the Act, although a good step forward, would have little impact on its own work. The Society's programme of financial grants to patients would not be affected because these were paid almost exclusively to patients at home. The only small relief to the Society's funds would be that patients' travel costs to hospitals for treatment would in future be met by the public authorities. Nevertheless, the passage of the Cancer Act represented a milestone in public policy and cancer. The Society's campaigning, stretching over a quarter of a century, had at last started to bring change.

Notes & References

1. One notable exception was the London County Council which during the 1930s, under the leadership of Herbert Morrison, built up local health services to provide 40,000 hospital beds – more than 70 per cent of the total available in the capital.
2. See *An Introduction to the Social History of Nursing,* by Robert Dingwall, Anne Marie Rafferty and Charles Webster, published by Routledge, 1988.
3. The Bible nurses became known as Ranyard nurses and they remained independent until they were incorporated into the district nursing service in 1965.
4. The progress of the planning application was recorded in the *Kentish Times* series, see editions of 22 April 1932, 27 May 1931, 23 June 1932 and 30 September 1932.
5. From the author's own knowledge, as recently as the 1980s local shopkeepers in another town in Kent objected to the development of a drop-in centre for cancer patients in the high street, on the grounds that its presence might distress and deter others, presumably shoppers, from the area.
6. Elliot's biographer, Sir Colin Coote, was very enthusiastic about the Cancer Act. A much decorated soldier of the First World War, Coote wrote in *A Companion of Honour* published by Collins in 1965, that 'the only sight worse than a fatal casualty from phosgene gas is the sight of a patient dying from one of the painful forms of cancer'.

5

Some Building Blocks

In the first twenty years of its existence, the Society had evolved from being chiefly a campaigning and proselytising pressure group, passionate but rather subjective in outlook and operating at the fringe, to an equally passionate but mainstream welfare charity, tackling a major social problem. From the early contempt of the medical establishment and indifference of public authorities, it was now earning not only the gratitude of those people with cancer it was able to help, but also the respect of all the agencies it worked with. This radically changed profile offered the Society the opportunity to grow and develop. A much broader range of people could now be attracted to the Society and encouraged to play a part in its work.

Although the Society had been founded in 1912 as a members' organisation, it was certainly not an open one. The first constitution said that the Society would consist of Patrons, Subscribing Members, Ordinary Members and Honorary Members, all of whom would be able to vote at the Society's general meetings. At an Annual General Meeting the members would elect both a general council and an executive council to run the day-to-day affairs of the Society. However, the 1912 document restricted membership to those with a recognised degree in a health-related subject, and to others with some special reason for wishing to join and who were also sponsored by two existing members. Applications for membership had then to be approved by the general council. These tight controls on membership were presumably intended to keep the Society within the influence of the founding fathers and true to their principles. They did not encourage wider participation. This had to change with registration as a benevolent society in 1924, and particularly if the Society was to attract much more widespread and popular support for its work.

Membership became open to 'Any person of British nationality … without regard to age, sex, occupation or residence.' New members still needed the approval of the general council, but membership could not be refused arbitrarily without the risk of falling foul of the Registrar of Friendly Societies. And in any event, the objective was now for the Society to recruit as many members as possible. The Society's publications increasingly gave emphasis to the recruitment of more members, and each existing member was encouraged to recruit six new members each year. The benefits of membership were advertised to include priority for personal care or assistance in case of need, use of the Society's collection of books about cancer, and 'letters of recommendation' (i.e. references) based on the amount subscribed to the Society.

This legal structure of a friendly society remained until the Society became a company limited by guarantee[1] in 1989, and it had an important influence on the organisation's character. In the simplest terms, friendly societies are run by their members and their rules must provide for this member control. The lay membership could maintain, in practice as well as in theory, a powerful role in the Society's affairs. Today, the structure of a friendly society is most often seen in co-operatives and housing associations, and in the few remaining workers' benevolent societies dating from Victorian times.

As has already been seen, the appointment of Reginald Gollop in 1930 to lead fund-raising was a great success. He was a skilled organiser and managed not just to increase the Society's membership, but also to galvanise the membership into more and more local activity. By

1934 the Society had official local representatives or voluntary visitors (often called almoners, as hospital social workers were known at the time) in over forty locations, and this number increased year by year until the Second World War. These locations formed the network for the growth of fund-raising activities, mostly organised as collections and public appeals. The membership register shows a concentration of members in many of these areas. Where local activity could sustain it, committees of the Society were formed. The first was in Bath, closely followed by Bolton, York, Cardiff, Heston & Isleworth, and Blackpool. The formation of new committees was approved by the Society and they were authorised to carry out the full range of the Society's activities – fund-raising, relief work and education.

In 1936 the Society published a suggested scheme for the organisation and administration of these committees. The recommended scheme rooted the committee in the local community and encouraged it to build relationships with doctors and hospitals, churches and local businesses, Rotarians and guilds, and educational establishments. The committees were often able to attract influential local people: the local Member of Parliament and his wife played leading roles on the Bolton committee; local councillors were active on the committees in Blackpool and York; clergymen, bank managers, doctors and retired military officers were often recruited, as well as prominent and charity-minded local ladies.

The committees raised funds. They funded directly the welfare payments to patients that would otherwise be administered through head office, and they gave support to their society visitors. They organised the distribution of clothing, bedding and even furniture that might be donated for the benefit of patients. Committees with local councillors as members would have an easy means of communication with the local authority. In York, the committee was able to open its own office.

The committees, although quite small in number, played a main stage role in the affairs of the Society at this time. The voluntary effort they contributed meant that the Society could make a much greater impact in these local areas. This helped to establish the Society's roots as a local or regional organisation, as well as a national one. The local committee was often the public face of the Society in its area of operation.

The growth of the Society could not, on the other hand, be wholly sustained by volunteers. Where possible, the Society did rely on voluntary workers, but the Society was becoming ambitious to meet the growing demand for financial support for patients. Shortly after the appointment of Gollop, and probably at his suggestion, the Society appointed a number of paid collectors. More than thirty were in place by early 1932, covering much of England.

The collectors were remunerated with a percentage of their takings. Later, a number of collectors were appointed as salaried organisers, and by 1936 organisers were employed to run collections and appeals in many parts of the country, including London, Kent, Liverpool, Yorkshire, East Anglia and the West Country. The performance of the organisers was reviewed quarterly by a finance committee set up by the executive committee to oversee and monitor income and expenditure. Organisers who failed to make a good enough return for the Society over and above their costs would not be retained. The Society was already acutely aware that the ratio of its costs to its income was an important measure of effectiveness, and a very visible one. The Society stressed in its reports that 'the highest possible percentage of revenue should be applied to the needs of those in distress'.

This was of course right in principle and the Society's lay members, at the council or in general meeting, would not hold back their criticism if they believed that costs were too high. Macmillan, on the other hand, understood that the basic administration costs of the Society were fixed, and that the lower the Society's income, the higher these costs would appear when expressed as a percentage. Moreover, administration costs included essential things like accounting and publicity and could not be reduced without putting the operations of the Society in jeopardy. The answer was not to cut into these basic administration costs, but rather to increase the income to the Society. This was a message he repeated regularly, though not always with success.

The Society's expansion also meant that a larger number of people had to be employed at the Society's head office. Voluntary helpers had long been used when available. Margaret Macmillan and many friends had provided the Society with its administrative support and fund-raising work from the Society's beginnings but they could no longer

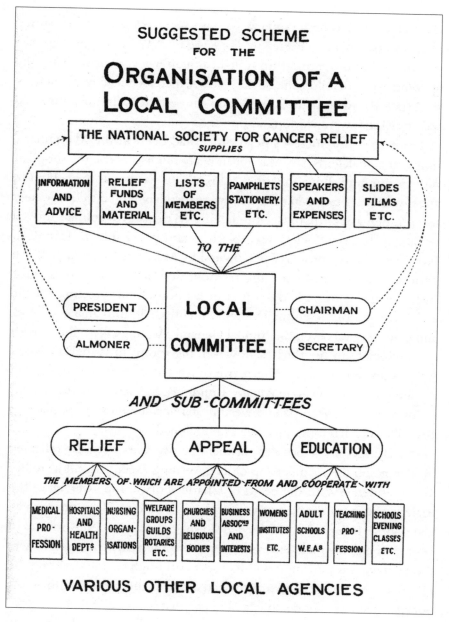

SUGGESTED SCHEME
FOR THE
ORGANISATION OF A
LOCAL COMMITTEE

THE NATIONAL SOCIETY FOR CANCER RELIEF
SUPPLIES

| INFORMATION AND ADVICE | RELIEF FUNDS AND MATERIAL | LISTS OF MEMBERS ETC. | PAMPHLETS STATIONERY. ETC. | SPEAKERS AND EXPENSES | SLIDES FILMS ETC. |

TO THE

PRESIDENT · · · · **LOCAL** · · · · CHAIRMAN

ALMONER · · · · **COMMITTEE** · · · · SECRETARY

AND SUB-COMMITTEES

RELIEF   APPEAL   EDUCATION

THE MEMBERS OF WHICH ARE APPOINTED FROM AND COOPERATE WITH

| MEDICAL PRO-FESSION | HOSPITALS AND HEALTH DEPTS | NURSING ORGAN-ISATIONS | WELFARE GROUPS GUILDS ROTARIES ETC. | CHURCHES AND RELIGIOUS BODIES | BUSINESS ASSOC^ns AND INTERESTS | WOMENS INSTITUTES ETC. | ADULT SCHOOLS W.E.A.s | TEACHING PRO-FESSION | SCHOOLS EVENING CLASSES ETC. |

VARIOUS OTHER LOCAL AGENCIES

How to organise a committee.

do it all. A part-time voluntary assistant secretary was first recruited from an advertisement posted in *The Times* in 1925, but the post-holder, Archibald Capern, retired from ill-health after a year or so. After the appointment of Gollop, the Society slowly increased its complement of paid staff. By 1938, apart from Gollop himself, five administrative and secretarial staff were working in London.

From 1912 the Society's head office had been in the Macmillans' house in Ranelagh Road. Macmillan really did live 'above the shop', or more accurately above the office. This arrangement was formalised in 1924 when two rooms in the house were formally rented to the Society for 10s. per week. In 1925 Douglas and Margaret Macmillan moved to Sidcup, but the Society was able to retain its tenancy in Ranelagh Road because the property was owned by Margaret Macmillan. It is a good indication of Macmillan's relationship with his Society that for its first thirteen years it was a part of his household. Meetings of the executive and of the council were frequently held in Ranelagh Road, and in leaner years even the Annual General Meetings. With the growth of the Society in the thirties, however, the rooms in Ranelagh Road were no longer adequate. Alternative office accommodation was found a couple of miles away in Albany Buildings, 47 Victoria Street, about midway between Victoria and Westminster and the move took place in 1935. The area has long since been redeveloped.

The changes in the Society between the two wars were also reflected by changes in the membership of its governing executive and its roll of vice presidents. With the death of Charles Forward in 1934, all of the early pioneers of the Society, apart from the Macmillans themselves, had gone. F. Higgins had succeeded Wilsher as treasurer. New intakes of council members included volunteers from the provincial areas where the Society was putting down its roots. Although strictly holding the office of vice chairman, Forward had acted as the chairman for most Society meetings. His death left a big gap that had to be filled.

The Society turned to finding a chairman from outside, and one who would add some distinction to the organisation. It chose Major General Joseph Cameron Rimington, a career soldier who had served with distinction in Turkey and India. He had cared for his wife dying with cancer and so brought his own poignant experience to the job.

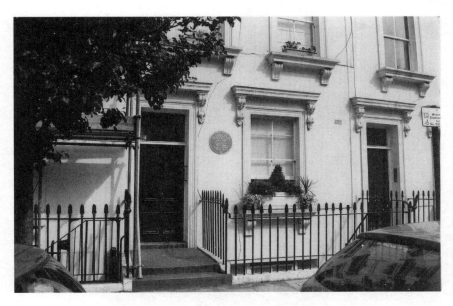

15 Ranelagh Road in Pimlico: home, office and campaign headquarters of the Society.

Rimington was elected in 1937 when he was 73 years of age. He was a conscientious chairman, attending all meetings of the Society and its committees, and frequently visiting the office in Victoria Street. It was a loss when, in 1942, he suddenly collapsed at a London bus stop and died. He was succeeded by a contemporary, Major General Lionel Charles Dunsterville, another veteran of the Empire's wars. Dunsterville had a particularly distinguished war record and was thought to be the model for Rudyard Kipling's character Stalky in the stories of Stalky & Co.[2] He played a full role at first, but his own health gave way and he died in 1946.

The other group of people associated with the Society were the president and vice presidents. The first post-holders had been appointed partly because of their position and status, but also because they shared the founders' views about medicine, medical research and vivisection. After the Society changed direction and began to grow it sought people of status and influence alone. The Countess Loreburn, wife of a former Lord Chancellor, became president in 1926, succeeded by Constance, Duchess of Westminster in 1935. In the same year, the ambassadors of Belgium, Brazil and Poland were included in the roll of vice presidents.

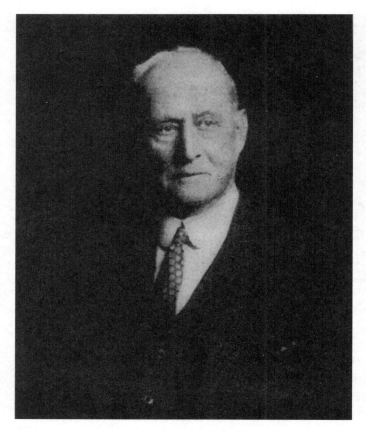

Major General Lionel Charles Dunsterville – 'Stalky'.

By 1938 there were thirty-eight vice presidents, including an archbishop and a bishop, one duchess, three marchionesses, three viscountesses – including Curzon and Halifax, two countesses, one baroness and eleven other titled ladies. Doubtless most of these people were names on a letterhead rather than active volunteers. However, the list is important because it demonstrated then, as it does now, how in a little more than a decade the Society had become solidly mainstream, widely accepted and supported, and with good links throughout society.

There were limits however. On 23 August 1939, Gollop wrote to the Home Secretary, Sir Samuel Hoare, seeking permission for the prefix 'Royal' to be added to the Society's name. Gollop had been urged to do this by a 'keen supporter', possibly one of the vice presidents. He argued in the letter that 'our work of mercy might be greatly increased and enhanced if the request were granted'.

Approval was not given, chiefly because the Society was still comparatively small. The civil servant dealing with the matter in the Home Office summed up the official view with:

> I understand it is a well meant endeavour but not one which stands at all high amongst medical charities. It ranks far below the Imperial Cancer Research Fund or the British Empire Cancer Campaign, neither of which has the title Royal.[3]

The request was probably a long shot and the response should not have been a great surprise. Royal recognition would come later.

Notes & References

1. A company limited by guarantee is a very common form for charities to take. It is similar to a commercial company, but the shareholders are replaced by members.
2. Dunsterville had been a schoolboy with Kipling at the United Services College at Westward Ho! in Devon.
3. See TNA file HO 144/21321.

6

Another War

At the end of the 1930s the Society could look back with some satisfaction on the past few years. All was going well. Income was rising, charitable work was expanding and the Society was becoming better known and more influential. For the first time, the Society's future seemed to be assured, at least for as long as cancer continued to damage and destroy lives. Then, on 3 September 1939, the Second World War began. It was a war that would last for nearly six years, bring devastation to many British cities, take over all facets of the British economy and involve almost every fibre of British society in a way that no conflict had ever done before. The war would inevitably have a major impact on the Society, as it surely would on every other voluntary organisation. Indeed, recalling the almost catastrophic effect that the First World War had had on the Society, Macmillan must have been acutely apprehensive to say the least about the Society's future when the conflict began. In the event, the Society's work was disrupted, the progress it had been making was slowed and in some ways reversed, and its all-important job of giving relief to people with cancer became more and more difficult to carry out. But at the same time, the Society was able to score some major achievements. Unlike in 1918, the Society emerged in 1945 with a strong base still intact, a record of achievement under wartime conditions and confident that it had a future role.

The first problem of wartime was that it became impossible for the Society to maintain its regular, internal communications or to hold its formal meetings. Douglas Macmillan was evacuated with his section of the Ministry of Agriculture to Lytham St Annes in Lancashire, more than 200 miles from the office in London. Chairman Rimington continued to live in London, and he was as assiduous as ever in regularly calling into the Society's offices and maintaining oversight of its affairs. Unfortunately, his successor Chairman Dunsterville lived in Devon. Other council and committee members were scattered all over the country. With the severe travel disruptions of wartime, it was decided to abandon most of the Society's formal meetings altogether, including even the Annual General Meetings. Decision-making had to be left to the honorary officers – the chairman, the treasurer and Macmillan – in communication with Gollop at the head office.

Although now located a full day's journey from London, Macmillan did not abandon his post of honorary secretary, but invited correspondence to him at his wartime address of 121 South Promenade. He also took advantage of his Lytham location by spending time visiting the Society's committees in the northern counties. At the same time, proper reporting, accounting and auditing of the Society's business continued, even if thrown temporarily out of gear. In the autumn of 1939 the Society published the only edition of its newsletter, *The Bulletin*, of the war years with the headline: 'The War Goes On'. The war it was referring to was not the war against Hitler, of course, but the war against cancer. It referred to the war 'against the pain and poverty with which many thousands of British cancer patients are afflicted' and explained that 'the oppressed whom we set out to succour are of all ages and of either sex – from the baby girl with cancer of the eyes to the old man who has no tongue'.

The important relief committee, which had been set up to consider in detail the growing number of applications for financial aid, was the one formal committee of the Society that continued to meet regularly and conscientiously. Macmillan was later to report that the committee's 'work has gone steadily on, without appreciable delay, month after month, and always steadily increasing ... [and that the committee] has won the approbation of Almoners and Doctors throughout the country and has brought the light of heaven into thousands of stricken homes'.[1]

In fact, the number of applications for relief fell in the first years of the war from 542 in 1939, down to 387 two years later. It then grew to a record 729 in 1944. Expenditure on support for patients was £9,131 (about £347,000 today) in 1939, and £13,380 in 1944. The fall in applications in the early years of the war coincided with the heavy bombing raids on London and other big cities, and the chaos and disruption that these caused.

The blitzes of London and of so many other cities and towns were yet an added blow to patients with cancer, whether they were being cared for in hospital or at home. Hospitals had to make provision for war casualties so there was pressure to discharge all but the most poorly of patients. The government's Emergency Medical Service required that all patients who were movable had to be evacuated to out-of-town hospitals or to makeshift hospitals converted from schools or other buildings. These could be far away from the patient's home, making visits from family difficult, if not impossible, in wartime conditions. Patients from St Thomas's Hospital at the foot of Westminster Bridge, for example, were transferred to Godalming in Surrey, some 30 miles away, and patients at nearby Guy's Hospital were sent to Tunbridge Wells or to Maidstone, also both 30 or more miles from London. From the London Hospital in the East End, patients travelled by ambulance or converted bus to Brentwood, Colchester or Southend. Similar arrangements were made for hospital patients in most of Britain's great cities. Only very sick patients remained but, worse for them, they had to face the possibility of bombing raids. Many of the big voluntary hospitals in London and elsewhere were hit by bombs, killing patients and staff, and very ill patients, to add to their sufferings, would have had to be moved to basement bomb shelters.

Being cared for at home was, potentially, just as horrendous. Medical and district nursing services were stretched to the limit with priority having to go to the victims of the war. At night ill patients would have to decide whether to stay in their beds at home and risk the air raids, or seek refuge in a public, and probably very basic, underground shelter. The prospect of becoming homeless, even temporarily, must have been a constant and over-bearing worry for people who were already quite ill. Emergency accommodation was inevitably communal, uncomfortable and lacking adequate facilities for privacy. The Society's visitor, Lilian Castle, who covered the area now known as Greater London reported that:

> 1940 was a very anxious year, as many patients lived in bombed districts, and it was many weeks, in some cases, before I could find them. Of my patients, 4 have lost their homes through enemy action, and 19 others have had their homes damaged. One patient ... died through enemy action. What a blessing the Society has been to them all in these troublous [*sic*] times.[2]

The war naturally affected the treatment that patients could receive. Radium was a dangerous material, and the possibility of an enemy bomb blasting the radioactive substance across the town or city was something to be avoided at all costs. Stocks of radium were therefore buried deep underground and only retrieved for patient treatment when safe to do so. In London a 50ft bore-hole was dug in Fulham, and some supplies of radium stored there. The stock of radium from the London Hospital was buried in a clay pit in Bedfordshire.

Deep X-ray therapy could be used as an alternative to radium, but the supply of equipment was limited. This supply was further depleted by the bomb damage to treatment facilities and operating theatres which was severe in many city hospitals. Westminster Hospital managed to get a programme of cancer treatment re-established after the Blitz in London, but at Guy's the radiotherapy department was completely destroyed by enemy action. Inevitably with wartime shortages, the hospitals could not meet anything like the needs of patients. Young doctors and nurses had been called up for active service so hospitals had to get by with far fewer qualified members of staff. The war must have prevented so many people with cancer from getting the curative or palliative treatments that they needed.[3]

Rationing, too, had an impact on the care and well-being of patients. The restrictions on the supply of foodstuffs meant that patients might not get the protein-rich diet or other foods they were recommended. The need for coupons to purchase clothes would have had implications for patients losing weight or needing extra warmth. The Society was able to purchase bulk supplies of blankets, sheets and cotton wool to alleviate some of the needs of patients with whom it had contact, but this was a small percentage of the number of people who had cancer. The privations of wartime, added to the shadowing burden of cancer, must have been an intolerable combination. It was surely no exaggeration when Macmillan described the work of the relief committee in this period as 'important, urgent and harrowing'.[4] Moreover, the unhappy truth was that despite all of the Society's efforts, it was able to do no more than a small fraction of what was needed. The Society's figures show that in 1944 a total of 1,278 people with cancer received some benefit from the Society in the form of a financial grant or a pension. In that year, the Society reported that 85,000 had died from cancer. Most people living with and dying from cancer would have received little relief, if any, at all.

The bombing war came as close as it could to the Society in the early morning of Wednesday 11 September 1940 when, thankfully long before office hours, Victoria Street was hit by high explosives. The Society's offices were severely damaged by the blast. Luckily, the Society's office equipment, records and stocks escaped destruction, but its main office in the building was no longer usable. Evacuation was considered, but Gollop and his staff, in keeping with the Londoners' spirit of defiance of those years, decided to remain in a smaller room for as long as possible. This was the middle of the Blitz, however, and travel to and from central London was becoming increasingly difficult. A second bomb exploded near to the Society's office a month later, and it was decided then to move office and staff to a safer locality. In due course, office space was found at 2 Cheam Court in Cheam, about 12 miles away in Surrey, and the Society's key operations were moved there in December 1940.[5] As it turned out, the outer London suburbs did not escape attack from the skies either, and Cheam Court was seriously damaged in the V2 raids later in the war. Luckily again, no one working for the Society was hurt.

The war did mean that the Society had to tighten its belt in many ways. The office in York was closed. The costs of stationery, postage and advertising increased, and large supplies of paper became hard to acquire. As well as the Society's newsletter being suspended, no other literature was produced. It became more difficult to raise funds by conventional means and for the sake of economy several paid organiser posts, including those in Devon, Hampshire, Kent and York, were dispensed with altogether. As a result of this contraction of activity and of the impact of the war generally, income fell between 1939 and 1941 from nearly £31,000 (about £1,180,000 today) to a little over £24,000 – a fall of more than 20 per cent.

Had this trend continued, the Society might well have emerged from the Second World War in a state as weakened as it had been in 1918. Luckily, that downward trend was arrested by the Society at last being allocated an appeal broadcast by the BBC Home Service (as BBC Radio 4 was called at the time). The BBC's offer to the Society to be *This Week's Good Cause*, came after many years of asking. Macmillan believed that the opportunity was given to the Society partly because of its growing reputation, but equally because of the influence and persistence of chairman Rimington.

The importance of BBC radio at this time cannot be underestimated. Television broadcasting had been discontinued for the duration of the war, and in any event very few people had television receivers in their homes. Radio, and the Home Service in particular, was the most important broadcasting medium in the country, providing the population at home with accurate information about the war and also with much of its popular entertainment. At times, incredibly, as much as half of the population was tuned into the BBC – more than 20 million people.

The Society's appeal was made on Sunday 28 December 1941 – a very good time when the number of listeners would have been high – by the Bishop of Bristol, the Right Reverend Clifford Woodward. The bishop's words were very poignant:

> The world is suffering on so vast a scale today that we are in danger of forgetting the suffering of individual men and women. But it is going on

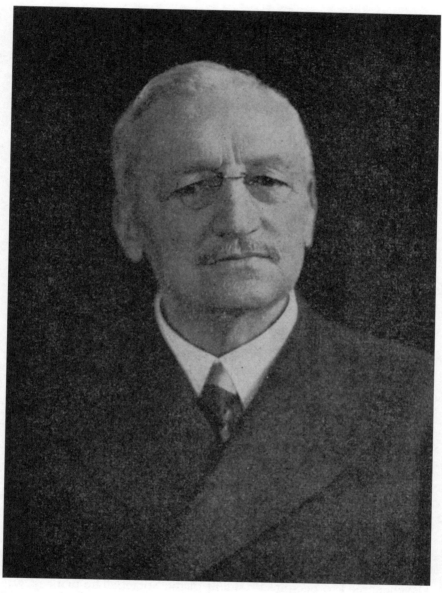

Major General Joseph Cameron Rimington, chairman of the Society, with his own personal reason for supporting cancer relief.

whether we remember it or not. There is, I suppose, hardly a street in any town in which there is not living at least one person in pretty constant pain. … I at least have seen enough of the terrible disease of cancer to know that I should dread more than anything, either for myself or for anyone I loved, the pain which nearly always accompanies it. I thank God for this Society, which exists to bring relief and comfort to its victims.

The bishop went on to explain how the Society's finances had been hit because of the war, and he prayed that the war would be brought to an end, but not 'at the expense of those who suffer, and whom in the past our gifts have done something to relieve'.

The bishop's words were very effective. More than £7,000 (well over £200,000 today) came flowing into the Society as a direct result of the appeal, a remarkable sum given the war context. Just as importantly, the appeal did something else. It raised the Society's profile and helped to sustain the income of the Society for the remainder of the war. In 1945 the Society's income for the year was £38,397.

The end of hostilities in 1945 brought to the Society an unexpected bonus of goods. The Red Cross had a large surplus of first aid and disaster relief supplies. It donated a stock of them to the Society, including 2,500lb of cotton wool, 11,000 bandages, 870 towels, 700 sheets and blankets, and quantities of dressing gowns, hot water bottles, bed pans and other pieces of equipment. The Society had no empty space of its own after the bombings, so a now redundant air-raid shelter was temporarily given over to the Society for storage and packing. The goods were parcelled by the Society's staff and sent to the Society's visitors, almoners and hospital outpatient departments for distribution to patients.

There was one other notable achievement during the war years. The Princess Victoria Battenberg, Dowager Marchioness of Milford Haven, agreed to become President of the Society. The princess was a granddaughter of Queen Victoria and the mother of Prince Louis, Supreme Allied Commander in Asia, who became Earl Mountbatten of Burma at the end of the war. The Imperial Cancer Research Fund had had royal patronage since its foundation. The Duke of York, who had become king in 1936, was the first patron of the British Empire Cancer Campaign. The appointment of the princess in 1940, albeit at the age

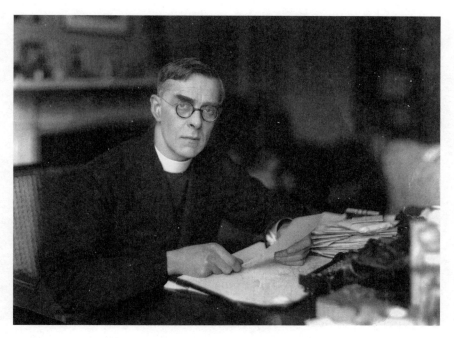

The Rt Revd Clifford Woodward, Bishop of Bristol: 'I thank God for this Society.'
(National Portrait Gallery)

of 77, established the first royal link with the Society. It must have done something to make up for the royal prefix disappointment of 1939.

The war years did give the Society, or at least Douglas Macmillan, the opportunity to ponder the future for the organisation, and to crystallise in his mind the postwar strategy and priorities. The Society's first priority after the war, Macmillan said, would have to be to 'maintain [and extend] the direct relief work which has brought such comfort into so many stricken homes'.

The second priority was home visiting, and Macmillan hoped to expand this considerably, most particularly in the poorer parts of the country. The third was the expansion of convalescent facilities for cancer patients, and the fourth, the provision of homes for people with cancer, particularly 'for those for whom there is no hope, and whose home circumstances offer them no cheer or comfort as they pass through the valley of the shadow'.

This was an important sentence, clarifying that the homes should be for the terminally ill. The word hospice was rarely used at this time and

it did not necessarily have the meaning it does today. There were very
few establishments in Britain that cared specifically for the dying, and
outside of London, none at all. Macmillan and the Society recognised
that the care of those dying with cancer was an area of utter neglect
and shortcoming. Using the statistics of war as a powerful point of
propaganda, Macmillan was able to say that despite the shocking toll of
Britons reported killed or missing as a result of enemy action – 446,000
– an even higher number, that of 481,000, died from cancer during
those years.[6]

The Society could as well reaffirm its commitment, not only to
cancer relief, but to better public information and education about the
disease. The war brought the British much closer to the people and to
the culture of the United States of America. Macmillan looked across
the Atlantic to what was happening there in cancer treatments and
care. The American Society for the Control of Cancer (later renamed
the American Cancer Society) had been founded just one year after
Macmillan's Society, but by the years of the Second World War it had
recruited thousands of volunteers to help with the work of cancer
prevention. It took a much more open, honest and forthright approach
than had ever been the way in Britain. Macmillan complained that no
organisation in Britain, apart from the Society, had attempted to tackle
cancer prevention through education. It was a theme the Society would
pick up a few years later and return to often. Meanwhile, the war had
brought about fundamental changes in British society and to people's
expectations for the future. A return to the pre-war systems of health
and welfare were inconceivable, particularly after the publication of the
Beveridge Report in 1942.[7] The popular will for change was reflected
when the first general election for ten years was held in 1945.

Notes & References

1. Report to a general meeting of the Society on 29 January 1946(2). *A Brief
   Report of the Work of the NSCR in the Three Years 1939, 1940 and 1941*, published
   by NSCR, 1942.
2. Ibid.

3. The number of people dying from cancer did increase during the war years, but not exceptionally. The reality for these times was that treatments were palliative rather than curative and so had only a limited impact on life expectancy.

4. *Cancer Relief in 1942, 1943 and 1944*, published by NSCR, 1945.

5. After the war, the main administration functions returned to the offices in Victoria Street, but the office at Cheam was retained to accommodate the patient welfare department.

6. Comparing the war dead with deaths from cancer had become a regular exercise for Macmillan. He used deaths from the Boer War and the First World War to make the same powerful point.

7. The Report on Social Insurance and Allied Services from Sir William Beveridge, commissioned by the government, recommended comprehensive state-operated social security to conquer, once and for all, the evils of illness, disease, ignorance, squalor and want. It was embraced as an election platform by the Labour Party.

7

Slow Progress

The landslide victory of the Labour Party in the postwar general election of 1945 was a landmark in British health and social policy. The public demand for a break with the past brought to power a government promising to introduce comprehensive health and welfare services, to be provided equally to all in accordance with their needs, and freely at the point of supply. Three major pieces of legislation[1] established the National Health Service, provided the National Insurance scheme to cover sickness, unemployment and pensions in old age, and introduced National Assistance as a safety net for people who fell outside the insurance scheme. The new health service was to provide care 'from the cradle to the grave', and the welfare legislation was to end, once and for all, the poverty and deprivation that had been, for many, the experience of the pre-war years. Or, at least, these were the expectations at the time.

A national health service had been recommended by the government's Inter-Departmental Committee on Social Insurance and Allied Services. This committee, chaired by William Beveridge,[2] published its report in 1942 with the robust declaration that there should be 'comprehensive health and rehabilitation services for prevention and cure of disease and restoration of capacity for work, available to all members of the community'.

Beveridge's report was not specific about how this service should be structured and funded, but the incoming Labour government was committed to implementing Beveridge's recommendations and the responsibility for this fell to the new Minister of Health, Aneurin Bevan.[3] Bevan was a firebrand Welsh socialist with a determination to bring social equality to the provision of health care in the UK. The organisation and the financial structure of the National Health Service were Bevan's creations with this principle of equality in mind. He wanted the NHS to be a single organisation responsible to the Minister with free and equal access to all, and he wanted it to be funded out of general taxation so that the better off paid most towards it.

The NHS came into operation on 5 July 1948. On that day the 1,771 municipal hospitals of England and Wales and the 1,334 voluntary hospitals were transferred to the NHS, and all medical general practitioners who opted in, and this was the vast majority, became contractors to the NHS. Patients needing medical treatment, no matter how poor or needy, were to receive it freely and on an equal basis to one another. This truly was a revolutionary break with the past. Never again would a citizen in need of medical attention have to do without that care because he or she could not afford the cost.

Potentially, the new NHS could have had a fundamental impact on the work of the Society. Although cancer was not mentioned specifically in the health legislation, the National Health Service Act of 1946 put a duty on the Minister of Health[4] to promote 'the establishment ... of a comprehensive health service designed to secure improvement in the physical and mental health of the people ... and the prevention, diagnosis and treatment of illness. ...'

If a comprehensive cancer treatment and care service were at last to be put in place, then the most important demands of the Society, including Douglas Macmillan's three hopes for the future, would have been met. The Society joined in the enthusiasm for this new direction of public policy and welcomed the National Health Service. Its report for 1946 said:

For thirty-five years this ... Society has maintained that the cancer problem, in many of its aspects, was one that the State itself should take in hand, and it is of great satisfaction to know that this overdue development is at last taking place ...

The new health service had to provide for its patients all dressings and appliances and all drugs, and local authorities now had to operate all ambulance services freely for patients. The Society would no longer be asked to give grants for these basic things. Local councils were given powers to do much more for sick and infirm people at home. As well as operating the district nursing service, they could provide equipment such as wheelchairs and commodes and domestic help services. Local councils could also provide for convalescence. Many of the additional powers to local authorities were again, like much pre-war legislation, permissive only. They did not place a duty on local authorities to provide these extra services, only the power to provide them if they wished to do so. The immediate impact of the new health service on the Society should have been to reduce the number of grant applications for these essential needs now supplied by the state, and indeed there was some nominal fall and some levelling off over the next couple of years. But within four years the trend began to move steadily up again. The welfare state just could not be all-embracing and its limits were becoming clearer.

The health service might now provide transport for patients to attend hospital for treatment, but it did not cover the costs of poor relations visiting a patient. Dressings and drugs were now provided freely, but not extra clothing or bedding. The costs of extra heating, better nourishment and other comforts could only rarely be met by the public authorities. There was a gap between what local councils had the power to provide for their residents and what they could afford to provide. To give just one example, the Society reported in 1949 that, 'Domestic help for poor invalids under the Act is still conspicuous by its absence, and even where it can be arranged the local authority often requires payment at rates quite impossible for the class of patients concerned'.

In fact, the late 1940s was a period of great austerity for the country and both national and local government expenditure was tightly restricted.

Britain was deeply in debt because of the war, much infrastructure in the country had been devastated by bombing, and unusually bad weather, among other things, hampered reconstruction. Rationing was still in place and utility was still the design feature for consumer goods. It was hardly surprising that the new welfare state could not provide a fully comprehensive range of health and social services, and that public authorities had to decide what should be the priorities.

The picture was much the same when it came to financial benefits for the sick and needy. National Assistance, which had replaced the Poor Law in making means-tested provision for those who fell through all the other welfare nets, operated at little more than subsistence level. Moreover, any support from the Society could even be included in calculating the means of a patient. In 1949 the Society reported:

National Assistance benefits are, in the majority of cases, very meagre indeed, doubtless because the officers administering them still work closely to scale. One is glad to find, here and there, officials who are prepared to 'use their discretion' and treat these poor sufferers with rather more generosity; but these are a minority, and only too often the Board's officials will 'restrict' the amount that the Society can pay to a patient by threatening to reduce their own contribution.

The Society was smart and responded to the bureaucratic parsimony of the National Assistance Board often by satisfying the patient's need directly, rather than through monetary contributions. Such gifts could not be taken into account when calculating a patient's means. Gifts of clothing, linen, food and many other things were organised for distribution. In 1949 a consignment of 500 food parcels was received from the people of Australia, all of which were sent on to the Society's poorest patients.

The austerity of these immediate postwar years did pass and Britain became a much more affluent place. Science and technology brought changes for the better to the way people lived their everyday lives. The Society always operated a flexible approach to its patient welfare work, meeting the particular needs of individual patients as far as it possibly could. As these times, fashions and expectations changed, so did

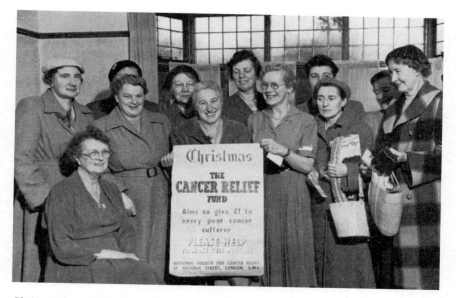

Christmas Appeal: £1 for every poor cancer sufferer.

the Society's scope of patient grants. Grants were made to pay for food liquidisers, radio and television rentals, toys and games for children, and even to pay for boarding expenses for pets. Of the more unusual grants, one was made to a patient for cattle cake so that he could continue to have fresh milk from his own cow. Another went to a poor and lonely man who was bought a budgerigar, complete with cage, because it was the one thing that would 'brighten his long days'. Patients who were overseas could be assisted with the costs of their passage home. At Christmas time, an extra payment was often made to all patients 'on the books' to give them a little extra comfort, happiness and peace of mind. According to the Society's report for 1961, 'Any case, however unusual, is readily considered and no genuine application, of course, is ever refused.'

One dilemma for the Society was whether to help patients who had apparently been treated successfully and cured of the disease. The Society agreed 'to take a liberal view of such cases, especially where the patient was suffering any disability that was attributable to ... cancer, or where there was any suggestion that lack of adequate care and nourishment might lead to a recurrence'.[5]

It is of interest that during this period the Society often had several patients who had been in receipt of benefit for many years. In 1950, for example, forty patients had been receiving help for more than ten years, three of them for eighteen years. Five years later, ninety-seven had been known for more than ten years, and four of them for more than twenty years. The Society had always insisted on medical certification of a diagnosis of cancer, so, unless the diagnosis had been wrong, which is of course possible, these patients must have been genuine long-term survivors of cancer.

The grants programme was also used to help patients in hospital. Television was by no means universal at this time, and television sets were then very expensive. A suggestion came that a television set in the men's oncology ward at the Hammersmith Hospital in west London would greatly uplift the spirits of the patients. The Society purchased and installed a set, and then did the same for Mount Vernon Hospital, the Hostel of God in Clapham, Lambeth Hospital and elsewhere. At Lambeth, the television was installed in the female radiotherapy ward which it was reported was for 'some 30 patients', and 'was nearly always well-filled'. The estimated cost of purchasing and installing a television in 1954 was £90 – the equivalent of more than £1,500 today – so these grants must have been very welcome.

For nearly thirty-five years after the end of the Second World War, the patient welfare programme continued to dominate the charitable work of the Society and its yearly expenditure. The amount of the Society's budget going towards patient welfare, in both cash terms and real terms, increased until 1970. By then, more than 10,000 people were being helped in this way every year. It was the growth of the Society's building and construction programme, with its emphasis on hospices, which finally shifted the balance of charitable expenditure away from patient grants during the 1970s. However, patient welfare continued to be one of the Society's most important charitable activities. Later, as will be seen, it evolved to take on a greater significance.

It had become clear pretty quickly to the Society that the NHS was not as comprehensive as its founders had perhaps intended or expected. In 1949, just one year after the new service had come into being, the Society was to report that:

Most distressing of all (to us, as well as to the smitten families) is the grievous absence of accommodation for cancer patients, discharged from hospital and needing the utmost care and attention, but having no relatives who are able to give it. Especially frequently does this arise in the case of elderly people. The State hospitals and therapy centres are doing magnificent work in the treatment of patients, by the most advanced methods, but there is not one Regional Board, from Cornwall to Caithness, that can yet provide adequate lodging (to say nothing of comforts) for the convalescent, the lonely and the dying.

It was somewhat unrealistic of the Society to expect everything in cancer treatment and care to be put right so soon after the NHS had taken responsibility. Indeed, one of the problems the new NHS had to cope with was the legacy of long-term neglect and war damage to the hospital infrastructure. However, the Society had reason to be impatient. It still regularly published the cancer mortality statistics for the country, which continued to show an ever increasingly upward trend. In 1946 the Society reprinted the official statistics to show that in the UK as a whole that year, 88,650 people had died from cancer. Three years later the number had increased to 94,000. Without health services to provide the special care that these patients needed, the cold statistics were the outward sign of a vast amount of suffering.

For cancer patients, what was left of the private and voluntary health sectors after the transfer to the NHS was just as unhelpful. A survey of some hundreds of private nursing homes, conducted by the Society in 1949, 'revealed that the majority of them are unable or unwilling to take cancer patients, and that where they are prepared to do so, the charges are, only too often, prohibitive. We have found a few worthy exceptions, but they are very few, and mostly very small.'

In 1951 the Society published *The Book of Cancer Relief* which included a list of private nursing homes that would care for patients with cancer. There were more than 100 homes on the list, and predominantly they were in southern England and in retirement areas. The introduction to the list gave warning that, apart from many homes not caring for 'incurables', as patients with terminal disease were often described, 'Some of the homes ... have felt obliged to limit their acceptances to

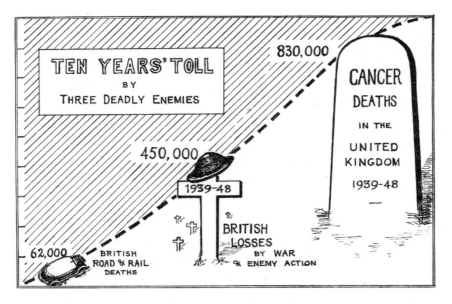

Statistics say it all.

patients with certain types of cancer (usually those that will not cause offence to other patients in the Home). ...'

The private nursing home sector chiefly catered for convalescence and for the fee-paying elderly. The only homes that welcomed the very ill and the dying were one or two early hospices run by orders of nuns. The Hostel of God, later renamed Trinity Hospice, in Clapham in south London, had opened in 1891, and St Joseph's Hospice in London's East End in 1905. The Society did continue to make grants to patients to cover the costs of convalescence in private nursing homes, but the amounts were quite modest although rising. In 1950 it was £674 (about £14,200 today), and ten years later it was £7,569.

The Society's commitment to provide its own homes for cancer patients had not been forgotten after the aborted attempt to use Park House in Sidcup. Macmillan and his colleagues were always looking out for suitable premises. In early 1952 a large house in Winchmore Hill in north London was inspected but rejected because of its general condition and location. The view now was that a home on the south coast would be preferable. Six months later, a property called The Manor House in Worthing on the West Sussex coast became available and a price of £10,000 was tentatively agreed before a surveyors report advised against it. Nursing homes came onto the market occasionally but usually these were only suitable for convalescent use. The Society was more concerned with providing homes that could be used for the terminally ill. Macmillan did not think it would be possible for the Society to build to its own design, and he was nervous of the local objections that had thwarted the Park House project.

An option was lost in Chislehurst because the Society could not bid in time, and a property in Sevenoaks was rejected because of its shabby condition. At last, but not until 1960, a property thought to be suitable was found in Southborough, a small district just to the north of Tunbridge Wells in Kent. The property, a rambling Victorian house called Helstonleigh, at 38 Pennington Road, was already in use as a nursing home and on the market for £7,500. This time, the surveyor's report was satisfactory and the purchase was completed.

Helstonleigh had the capacity to accommodate up to twelve patients. As a general and non-specialist nursing home it was not really suitable for the care of the dying, although it is not clear that this was understood at the time. The patients were all to come from the local area, and medical care was to be provided by the patients' general practitioners.

At the beginning the Society found it difficult to recruit a matron or sufficient staff to run the home, and consequently the home had to operate below its capacity. A matron was finally appointed but she proved to be unsatisfactory, and in November 1961 the home had to be closed for a short period. The three patients remaining were transferred to other nursing homes. The home re-opened in the new year, but then had to close again eighteen months later for repairs and alterations. On completion of the works, the home could only be licensed to care for nine patients, and as an average it looked after only five at any time. With operating costs of £7,000 per annum, Helstonleigh was hopelessly uneconomic. The Society decided to close the home and its patients were transferred to a nursing home in Hastings in October 1964.[6]

The nursing home project had always been experimental, and had it been successful Helstonleigh might have been the first of many Society homes around the country. However, the project had been a

failure from which the Society learned many lessons. The first was that
to be financially viable, a nursing home for the very ill had to have a
much greater capacity, and that small converted houses rarely provided
the ideal infrastructure. The second lesson, and probably the more
important one, was that the Society just did not have the skills, expertise,
or management structures to operate homes for inpatients. The Society
would not again attempt to directly operate and manage its own homes
for cancer patients.

Although the programme of patient welfare was still, at this time,
dominating the Society's expenditure, it certainly did not exclude
all other activity. For Douglas Macmillan the work of education and
spreading information was just as important. He was somewhat gratified
with an article by Dr Percy Stocks, the chief medical statistician at the
General Registry, which appeared in the *News Chronicle* in 1947 and
which concluded that geographical factors played a part in cancer
causation and suggested that climate and sunshine and water supply
were among them. This appeared to support the thrust of the Society's
'blue book' published some thirty years before, although the conclusions
would again turn out to be spurious.

A considerable amount of information and intelligence was published
in *The Book of Cancer Relief*, already referred to. It was priced at 2s.
6d. a copy (i.e. 12.5p, about £2.50 today) and 1,500 copies were sold
between July and October 1951. Most of the articles had been written
by Macmillan. There was one describing cancer and the process of cell
division, one about treatments and another about symptoms. There
was a glossary of medical terms, warnings about 'quackery' and many
references to cancer research. Macmillan had lost much of the antipathy
to cancer research he had expressed a quarter of a century or more
before, and even spoke well of his old bête noire Ernest Bashford.

The booklet was intended to throw light on cancer and to make it
more understandable and less fearsome to the average person in the
street. At the time the subject of cancer was still cloaked in darkness
and secrecy. It was common practice for diagnoses of cancer to be
withheld from patients and their close families because of the fear and
distress that this would bring, and the Society's own welfare grants were
usually given to patients anonymously to hide the words 'cancer relief'.

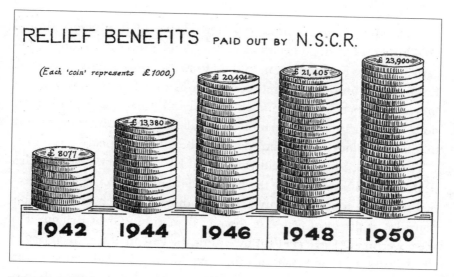

From *The Book of Cancer Relief.*

Yet, it was still clear to Macmillan that if people lived in such fear of cancer they would be much less likely to seek medical attention on the appearance of early symptoms.

In the chapter headed 'The People Want To Know', Macmillan argued for a much more open and frank discussion about cancer, following the lead from the American Cancer Society. Macmillan agreed that he was at one with the leading surgeon Lord Moynihan who, when opening the radium institute in Liverpool before the war, had said:

> I am convinced that further progress in the direction of curable cancer will only occur when we take the public into our confidence. I have been told that my advocacy of enlightening the public on the disease will only have the result of frightening them to death. On the contrary, I am sure my advocacy will frighten people to life!

The plea for more openness would not be heard for some decades yet. A footnote in *The Book of Cancer Relief* reported that the Minister of Health's Cancer and Radiotherapy Advisory Committee (predominantly a doctor-led body) had just told the minister that it would be undesirable for any cancer publicity to be directed at the general public. The committee preferred that such publicity should only be spread through health professionals. The subject was debated in parliament the following year. In the House of Lords[7] a retired surgeon, Lord Webb-Johnson, insisted that as far as cancer was concerned, it 'never did a patient any good to be told and it had almost invariably done serious harm by undermining morale. In my ... career I met only one strong-minded man who wanted to be told the worst.'

This was a commonly held view and it has to be acknowledged that in the United States, where the work of The American Cancer Society had spread so much publicity about the disease, twice as many people named it as the most feared of diseases than did in Great Britain.[8] For the government Patricia Hornsby-Smith, the Parliamentary Secretary to the Minister of Health, said that there was 'deeply divided opinion from responsible medical quarters' and that she feared that more publicity about cancer would cause distress and public alarm, and that 'consulting rooms would be swamped with frightened people, and that overworked GPs would have more work thrown upon them'.

The junior minister also expressed her worry that the demand for hospital beds would increase and that an intolerable burden would be placed on existing resources.[9] This seems to have been a rare, but honest, admission from government that if all people with cancer received early diagnosis and sought treatment, the National Health Service would be unable to cope.

Many more tracts from the Society about cancer followed the 1951 booklet. A series of education leaflets was produced taking forward the themes of prevention, symptoms and cures. Of particular interest now is the attention the Society gave to smoking. Macmillan had been staunchly against tobacco for all of his life, and the potential dangers of the habit had been raised in the Society's early literature. In the early fifties, several studies by Richard Doll and Bradford Hill pointed to smoking as the direct cause of lung cancer. Surprisingly, however, these studies were played down by many, including the Ministry of Health. Even the Cancer and Radiotherapy Advisory Council sought to qualify the findings by saying that there was still no certain evidence that tobacco smoke contained carcinogens and that it was unlikely the increase in lung cancer was entirely due to smoking.[10] The Society pointed out that deaths from lung cancers had increased eight-fold for men in the thirty years up to 1953, and that one-third of male patients receiving relief from the Society had been diagnosed with lung cancer. In a battle cry the Society declared in its report for 1957:

> Let these figures be clearly grasped: 20,000 painful deaths from this one form of cancer alone. … And all this, or most of it, the result of a costly and needless drugging habit increasingly indulged in by men, women and even children.

The Society published the leaflet *Is Smoking Worth While?* and made special efforts to distribute it to schools, colleges and youth associations. But it was a decade or more before the link between smoking and cancer was widely accepted, and meanwhile lung cancer mortality continued its exponential rise. On several occasions the Society drew attention to the financial support given by the tobacco companies to the Medical Research Council – support that would be regarded as quite unethical today.

One other area of the Society's work needs to be discussed, albeit briefly, and this is, perhaps surprisingly, research. Strictly, the Society had given up any role in research back in 1924, and its publications often explained this and directed any research interest to the British Empire Cancer Campaign. However, the Society continued to receive gifts, and particularly legacies, with the donors' instructions that they were to be used for research.

In 1946 a substantial legacy of £2,600 (worth about £66,000 today) had been received from a Miss Morrison of Edinburgh. The Society decided that it would retain the sum as a capital endowment and use the annual income for research. The Society also decided that it would support specific areas of research rather than merely pass the income to a cancer research charity. The first grant was made to the Christie Hospital to support research into the optimum dosages of radiotherapy for the treatment of various cancers. This helped to set for the Society its research parameters. It would support research into treatments and care, but not into the causes of cancer which was reserved for the research charities, and this exclusion remains in the charity's constitution to

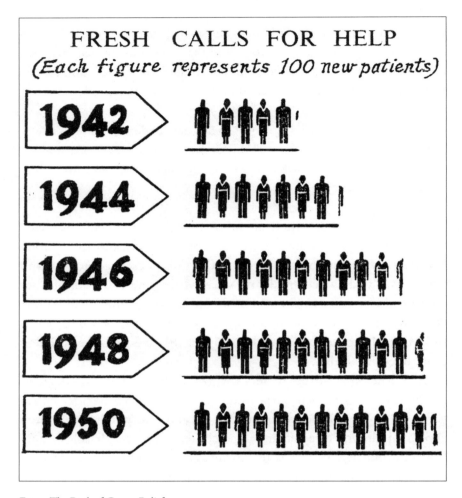

FRESH CALLS FOR HELP
(*Each figure represents 100 new patients*)

1942

1944

1946

1948

1950

From *The Book of Cancer Relief*.

this day. One project given support was an enquiry into the prevalence and nature of smoking habits among school children in Oxfordshire. Another, though of less certain value, was support for a survey in 1957 of cancer clinics in the United States by the Revd Brian Hession. Hession, a smoker, had had surgery in the States for lung cancer and the outcome appeared promising. He believed that American treatment techniques were superior to those in Britain and he wrote a book about his experiences called *Determined to Live*. In 1961, sadly but inevitably for the time, he succumbed to the disease.

Notes & References

1. The National Health Service Act 1946, the National Insurance Act 1946, and the National Assistance Act 1948.

2. Beveridge (1879–1963) was an economist and social reformer with a prestigious record as an academic and public servant. He was briefly Liberal Member of Parliament for Berwick-upon-Tweed before becoming Baron Beveridge and leading his party in the House of Lords.

3. Bevan (1897–1960) worked as a miner before becoming Labour Member of Parliament for Ebbw Vale in south Wales. He resigned from the Labour government in 1951 after the decision to impose charges on NHS prescriptions, spectacles and dental care.

4. The National Health Service (Scotland) Act 1947 put a similar duty on the Secretary of State for Scotland.

5. Minutes of Annual General Meeting, 15 March 1939.

6. Helstonleigh was later demolished and a block of apartments for the retired now stands on the site.

7. Debate, 13 May 1952.

8. In polls conducted by the Gallup Organisation in 1949, 57 per cent of US respondents named cancer as the disease that they feared the most compared with 29 per cent in Great Britain.

9. Debate, House of Commons, 23 July 1952.

10. The chairman of the committee, Sir Ernest Rock Carling, a most eminent surgeon and radiologist, famously said, 'I have smoked all my life and have no intention of giving it up.'

8

More Building Blocks

The twenty years that followed the Second World War saw the Society's income steadily grow. The one exceptional year was 1947, when Britain froze up in the worst winter weather for decades and when all belts were tightened. But, overall the Society's income increased from its base in 1945 of £17,362 (about £460,000 today),[1] to £94,910 ten years later, and to £315,257 (nearly £4 million today) in 1965. The Society was, more or less, tripling its size every ten years. This was not rapid growth by any means but it was a gradual and solid progression. The Society's membership also grew steadily from 627 in 1947 to 3,649 by 1965. Very importantly, in 1960, the Society could boast that it had 164 local committees or voluntary representatives, compared with the mere handful of fifteen years before. These were now in every large city and town of England, Scotland and Wales, and with one in Belfast. The reach of the Society had at last become national, in reality as well as in name.

A major contributor to this growth was Frank Georgeson. New local organisers had been employed to replace those lost with the outbreak

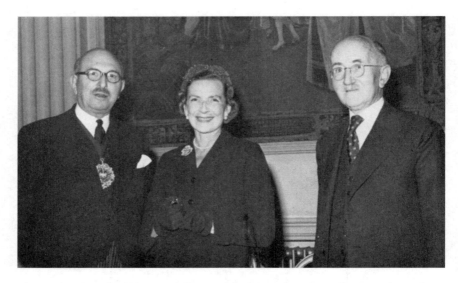

The Lord Mayor of London, Sir Cullum Welch, the Countess Mountbatten and Douglas Macmillan at the reception at Mansion House in 1957.

of war, although a shortage of good staff was a universal problem. Georgeson, who had been appointed organiser for Lancashire, was so effective that he was asked to move to London to take over fund-raising organisation on a bigger scale. In the tradition of Reginald Gollop,[2] Georgeson brought about a big expansion of local voluntary activity which was the driver for much of the increasing income. He had a great deal of organising zeal. He wrote to the mayors of major cities and towns where Society activity was low, encouraging them to start committees of the Society as a permanent legacy of their mayoralty. Many obliged. In 1957 even the Lord Mayor of London helped by holding an 'At Home' at the Mansion House for 200 or more friends and supporters of the Society.

The growth of local voluntary effort brought forward much new initiative. The Society's local activists had mainly used the traditional forms of fund-raising. Collecting boxes left in shops, pubs and other key locations, street collections – often called flag days – and house-to-house collections were still the mainstays of income generation. But, new ideas followed. Collections of 'widows' mites' became a popular fund-raising idea, particularly in the lean years of the immediate postwar period. At the other end of the spectrum, the Bridlington Committee held a 'Spring Fayre' in 1949 that earned a profit of £1,900 (about £42,000 today). The event was opened by Dame Sybil Thorndyke, the very famous actress of the time. It became a regular event, with the following year's fayre, opened by the Earl of Halifax, making a profit of £2,000.

Another famous actress, Hermione Gingold, opened a big event for the Society in London's Battersea Park; a marbles tournament was held in Castleford; a 'tramps' ball' in Eltham; an art exhibition was put on at the Tea Centre in London; collections were held in all of London Transport's bus garages; students at Aberdeen University made 'Cancer Relief' their rag charity; and the National Operatic and Dramatic Society used its diamond jubilee year celebrations to support the Society. At Cowdray Park in West Sussex a collection was held during a polo match where the star player was Earl Mountbatten of Burma. In 1957 the Duke and Duchess of Roxburghe first opened their home, Floors Castle at Kelso in the Borders, to visitors to raise funds for the Society and some thousands of people crossed their gates raising £1,300 (about £20,000 today). In addition to jumble and 'bring and buy' sales, the Society sold its own Christmas cards and its own pens embossed with the Society's initials NSCR. Charity shops in Victoria and Oxford Street were opened for the Christmas shopping period. Local committees held a determination and a spirit of competition to be among the most successful of money-raisers, and the Society began to publish each year in its newsletter a list of committees with their respective fund-raising performance.

The Society had a compelling cause. Its yearly reports and fund-raising literature made use of countless patient case histories to demonstrate the value of its work and the impact the Society had on the lives of so many unfortunate people. The Society declared that before its existence, 'Many thousands of Britain's victims of this cruel affliction, suffered also from poverty, neglect and lack of comforts' and that 'not a single valid case has ever been refused help'.

The Society began a scheme to 'adopt a patient', long before charities working in overseas aid used the idea. Members and supporters were asked to make regular donations to help, or to sponsor, particular patients.

The Society even placed advertisements in newspapers containing brief histories of patients or their families and inviting donations to support them. The identities of both patients and donors were kept in confidence from each other, but the scheme still gave donors the added pleasure of knowing exactly how their gift was being used. One newspaper advertisement placed by the Society was for a

> *Cancer sufferer, poor old man (72), is in need of special diet of eggs, meat extracts etc. which he cannot afford. Please help us to care for him.*

The newspaper in question somehow made its way across the Atlantic and the Society reported, with some amazement, that it received on the old man's behalf, from a resident of the town of South Orange in the US state of New Jersey, 'a most exciting parcel of foods (including a dozen eggs which unfortunately travelled badly!)'.

It was during this period that a new motto appeared, and one more in keeping with the Society's welfare work. For inspiration, the Society turned again to its founder and adopted the motto of the Highland Clan Macmillan – Miseris Succurrere Disco. These words of Latin are by Virgil and from his epic poem, The Aeneid. The modern translation, according to Sir Kenneth Calman, 'I learn to look after those in need', still has much relevance for the organisation, and even more so as it has expanded into medicine, nursing and other aspects of cancer and palliative care. Improving the lives of people with cancer is only possible through continuous learning.

The growth and development of the Society's national and local fund-raising activity and of its welfare work helped to boost the income received from legacies. Douglas Macmillan had always encouraged people to think about the Society when they wrote their wills and the Society's annual reports had always included advice about the correct terms to use in their drafting. In the early days of the Society one or two legacies of significant size had helped to keep the organisation afloat. On several occasions, income to the Society from legacies had more than outstripped all other income, sometimes by a considerable extent. In 1945 the income from legacies was £4,353 (about £115,000 today) and it represented about one-quarter of all income. In 1955 income from legacies was £40,630 and it represented more than 40 per cent of all income. By 1960 the income from legacies was £134,959 (about £1,910,000 today) and it had risen to more than half of all income. The Society, like many other charities, had become reliant on legacies to support a major part of its charitable work. However, the number of bequests a charity may receive in a year, and their monetary value, are inevitably subject to much fluctuation. The maintenance of all the other fund-raising activities was absolutely crucial.

After the considerable success of the wartime radio appeal, the Society had tried again to get onto the air waves. It was successful in 1948. The Revd Leslie Weatherhead, one of the leading non-conformist churchmen of the day made the appeal with a religious fervour that might have come from the young Douglas Macmillan himself. He said that:

> Jesus Christ called one disease the work of Satan. I am sure that is how He would describe cancer. Let us never regard it as the will of God. The will of God is that we should fight it with all our powers, banish it, as in this country we have banished plague ...

The Reverend's polemic was effective and the appeal raised about £6,300 (about £141,000 today). This was getting on towards being one-fifth of the Society's income for the year, and so a very major boost indeed. A further radio broadcast was offered in 1959, and this time it was made by the TV and radio personality Miss Barbara Kelly. The Society had always appreciated the value of celebrities supporting its work and it had been able to attract many big names. In addition to Sybil Thorndyke and Barbara Kelly, the Society had recruited the famous footballer Stanley Matthews, the actresses Vivien Leigh and Celia Johnson, socialites Sir Bernard and Lady Docker, and singer Gracie Fields, who even paid a visit to the Society's head office. The comedian Arthur Askey was also a regular supporter of the Society, doubtless persuaded to help by his sister Irene, who was employed as a member of the Society's fund-raising appeals team.

Of course, not all fund-raising initiatives came with great promise. In 1952 the Society experimented with house-to-house collections of

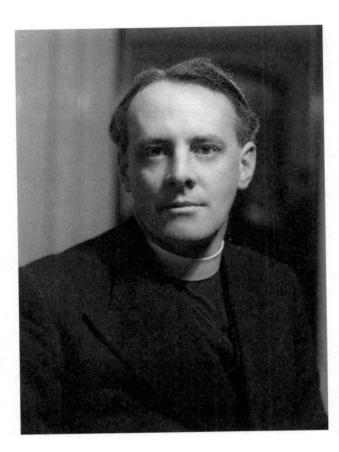

The Revd Leslie
Weatherhead: 'the
will of God is that we
should fight [cancer]
with all our powers.'
(National Portrait
Gallery)

salvage – doubtless a euphemism for 'rags and bones' – but of the men
offering to do this work 'most of them appeared to be undesirable'.
One man in Slough 'seemed to be a superior type', but the scheme
was dropped after complaints were received from the public and the
Society feared that its good name might be tarnished. One of the
more bizarre proposals was from an American would-be film producer,
Mr Norman Ranco, who was seeking finance for a futuristic film to be
called *The Electronic Doctor*. The plot included the discovery of a cure
for cancer and in return for putting up some of the cash needed to
make the film, the Society would have received the profits from the
box office. The Society wisely declined the offer and, not surprisingly,
there is no record of Mr Ranco ever completing his film. Yet another
American offered to exhibit for the Society his 'unique work of unusual

art', which was a replica of the Eiffel Tower made out of 125,000 tooth picks. He planned to bring the 16.5ft model from New York to England on the *Queen Mary* and asked only for the Society to fund his return passage. Again, the Society politely said no.

The Society took a great deal of pride in the voluntary effort that underpinned much of its fund-raising and it could be almost disparaging about other charities which had chosen a different balance between paid staff and volunteers. The 1960 report boasted that the Society 'does not employ professional (and expensive) organisers to amass huge funds for its work, but prefers to encourage, by quieter means, the sympathy and support of understanding people'.

This tended to be Douglas Macmillan's own style, which had been impressed upon the Society too. It differentiated the Society from many other growing charities. Looking closely at the percentage of income spent on charitable work was a regular exercise. The Society's governing council by now consisted of many representatives of the local voluntary committees and they did not expect to see larger amounts allocated to management and administration costs. For much of the period under discussion, about three-quarters of the Society's annual income was spent on its charitable work, and great efforts were made to squeeze other costs. The charitable work could not be performed without some cost. As the Society had already reported, 'The relief work of the society continues to increase and this necessitates increasing expenditure for wages, postages, equipment, rent and other services'.[3]

The Society was evidently concerned about criticism, or potential criticism, of its costs compared with those of other charities and added a warning to readers that: 'It should be noted that certain other fund-raising organisations, which claim to operate at a much lower cost-ratio, omit to make clear the nature of their administrations.'

The point that the Society was trying to put across, although not at all clearly, was that the Society's charitable expenditure all went to benefit patients. By contrast, other charities – and the British Empire Cancer Campaign might have been in mind – made charitable grants to other bodies which also had administration costs to carry. So, a fair comparison with the Society was not possible unless the costs of both grant giver and grant receiver were lumped together. It was a good, if rather negative, point to make.

These years of gradual growth and development, and of adaptation to the postwar era, were also years with many endings. The Society's first royal president, Princess Victoria Battenberg, died in 1950. Although she had been too elderly to play an active part in the Society's life, she was always supportive and helpful. A family link was maintained when shortly after her death her daughter-in-law, the Countess Mountbatten of Burma, agreed to take on the Society's presidency. Edwina Mountbatten, wife of the king's cousin and former Supreme Allied Commander in Asia and last Viceroy of India, already had several long-standing commitments to charities and she was known to be very conscientious in undertaking work for them. It was, therefore, something of a triumph for the Society to get her support. She took the role of president seriously, and played her part both attending important events and sending messages of encouragement when she was not able to. The countess died early in 1960 while on an overseas trip for another charity. Gollop, the Society's first employee who had done so much to kick-start the organisation in the inter-war years, left the Society on sick leave in 1950 and died the following year. His illness, not diagnosed in its early stages, turned out to be cancer. The Society also saw a milestone pass in December 1957 when Margaret Macmillan, the founder's wife, died after a long and unhappy illness at the age of 89. She had helped to sustain the Society, as well as her husband, for more than forty years.

Douglas Macmillan married again the following year. His second wife, Nora Owen, worked for the Society as the assistant secretary. But by this time, he too was beginning to slow. From his office of honorary secretary, he had become chairman of the Society in 1949.[4] Since his retirement from the civil service in 1946 he had devoted a greater part of his time to the affairs of the Society. Attending the office in Victoria Street almost daily, Macmillan was in effect an executive chairman. He worked from an old, roll-top desk and looked after much of the Society's administration. This allowed secretary Georgeson to travel widely, setting up and nurturing the local fund-raising organisation. Ill-health began to affect Macmillan in 1958 when he was 74 years old; he continued in his office for another five years, although he could attend fewer and fewer meetings. In 1962 his health further deteriorated and in September 1963 Macmillan decided to retire from all Society work. He wrote formally to the secretary:

> The time has now come when I must submit my formal resignation as Chairman of this Society.
>
> As you are already aware, I have not been able, owing to illness and advancing years, to take any effective part in the work or supervision of the Society during the current year, and it is now quite clear that I cannot contemplate any resumption of those services. My interest in cancer, and in the relief and comfort of its victims, has persisted for well over half a century now, and though that interest still continues, I find myself (in my 80th year) too tired, mentally and physically, for any useful effort. I therefore lay down my former responsibilities for some more competent person to take up.

To mark Douglas Macmillan's extraordinary contribution to the Society, a portrait of him in oils was commissioned from the accomplished painter R.R. Tomlinson of the Royal Academy. It was presented to him at the Society's Annual General Meeting on 10 November 1964.[5] Douglas and Nora Macmillan moved to a house called Carylande in Castle Cary the following year. Nora became a member of the Society's council, allowing Douglas to keep in close touch with the Society's affairs, but he no longer had any part to play.[6] He died from cancer on 9 January 1969.[7]

It could be argued, and indeed it was, that Macmillan stayed too long at the head of his Society and that his influence stunted the Society's development. Certainly Macmillan was the most powerful influence in the affairs of the Society from 1911 until his retirement as chairman. He was responsible for appointing the key members of staff. He proposed those who held the important positions of trustees, treasurer and executive members, and mostly they were old friends and colleagues, or relations. No important decisions, and indeed few less important ones, were ever taken without Macmillan's participation in the process and his agreement with the outcome. The Society was

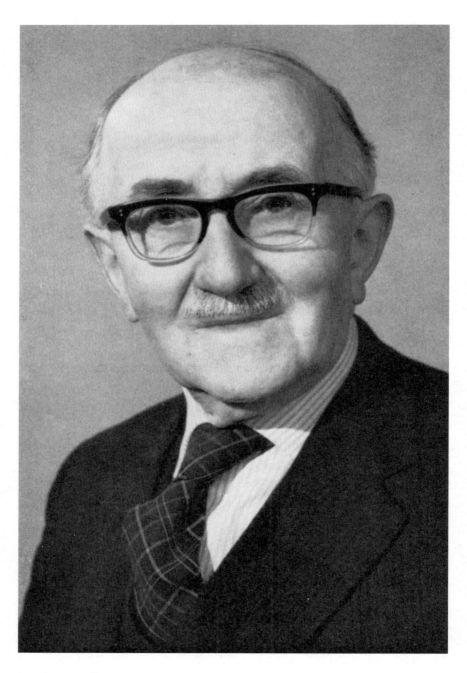

Douglas Macmillan in 1965.

sometimes accused of being a 'one man band', and it is beyond doubt that it would have been very difficult, if not impossible, for any initiative with which Macmillan disapproved to have gone ahead.

The records of meetings demonstrate the near reverence with which he was regarded. This must have made it very hard for other flowers to blossom. At the same time, Macmillan was a Victorian and an Edwardian, and he must have become increasingly dated as the postwar years passed by. Macmillan was not unaware of his critics, but neither was he particularly sympathetic to their points. At the Society's Annual Meeting in 1953 he faced them and said:

> I understand that certain individuals, possibly somewhat jealous or ill-disposed, have rather sneeringly called this a one-man society. There is perhaps an element of truth in this, but only to the extent that there is only one man who has been in it from its inception over 40 years ago, who has known all its strivings and difficulties, rejoiced in the progress of its great benevolent work, striven for its integrity of purpose and administration, and in general guided its steps. But there has been no dictatorship.

Macmillan then went on to stress the role and importance of the council elected by the Society's membership. But then he looked to his own retirement and pleaded for what might come after. He said:

> In any case the term of one person's active influence is limited, no doubt wisely, by the laws of nature and the time cannot be far distant when the responsibility for this great 'cause' will have to be borne by other shoulders. ...
>
> As the society becomes more and more influential, and possibly wealthy ... there will be people who will seek to get a hold upon it – not in the interests of our patients, but of themselves and their friends. The one thing I would beg of you is to oppose any such attempts to the utmost. ... I am sure that by prayer and care, such dangers can be thwarted and the integrity of the Founders' policies maintained.

It is very common, and indeed entirely understandable, for the founding father of an organisation to regard it as his own – almost as his own child.

And just as many parents find it difficult to let go, Douglas Macmillan cannot be criticised for a similar emotion.

Douglas Macmillan never received official recognition for his work in cancer care during his lifetime. He was awarded the MBE during the Second World War but this was for his help and support towards his young colleagues in the civil service. A self-effacing and very proper man he would never have sought reward or honour. Moreover, the controversial stands he had taken in his younger years would not have helped his case. He was a man of the highest morality, commitment, tenacity and determination, and a man with the deepest of compassion for the suffering of his fellow man. Without this mixture, it is most unlikely that the Society would have survived beyond its first big test. Macmillan wrote in the Society's report for 1959 words to describe the growth of his Society. He said:

> So the tiny seed, planted in Christian faith, watered and nurtured by countless gracious souls, has yielded the promised increase. To God be the Glory.

Macmillan had done much more than just plant the seed. He had done a greater part of the nurturing for more than fifty years.

He wrote a poem more than thirty years before his death which surely summarised his approach to life.

> *We are writing each one in the book of our life,*
> *A record of good or ill.*
> *And the fair, fresh days as they come to us*
> *Are pages we each must fill.*
> *Let the deeds we do and the words we speak*
> *Be tender and pure and true,*
> *That at least when we come to the story's end*
> *The book may bear reading through.*

Notes & References

1. To make some comparisons with other cancer charities, the expenditure of the Imperial Cancer Research Fund in 1947 was £27,828, and that of the British Empire Campaign was £130,000.
2. Gollop had become general secretary of the Society with the outbreak of war and so had taken on much wider responsibilities. In due course Georgeson would also be appointed to this post.
3. Report for 1958.
4. After chairman Dunsterville's death in 1946, Lord Darwen of Heys-in-Bowland became chairman until he was appointed a lord-in-waiting in 1948.
5. The portrait now hangs in the boardroom of the UK office of Macmillan Cancer Relief.
6. Macmillan was elected as president of the Society on his retirement as chairman, but he relinquished this post too in 1966.
7. Mrs Violet Brewser, Macmillan's niece, said in an interview in the late 1990s that all of Macmillan's seven siblings also had cancer during their lifetimes.

9

A New Era Begins

The new chairman chosen to fill the substantial gap left by Douglas Macmillan was the Duchess of Roxburghe. She had first become involved with the Society in the mid-1950s when she became president of the Society's Glasgow committee. She soon became a prominent supporter north of the border and then extended her activity southwards. As chairman she was hardworking and conscientious, rarely failing to attend the regular meetings in London even though some would have meant a 350-mile journey from Kelso. Macmillan had bequeathed to his successor a chairmanship that was executive in nature and the duchess had little choice but to play this role. She did so with some success.

Born Elisabeth McConnel, the duchess was from a Scottish Borders family. She married the 9th duke in 1954, but he would die twenty years later at the age of 61. In 1976 she married the Society's treasurer, the distinguished banker Jocelyn Hambro. The duchess was ambitious for the Society and saw that it had the resources and the standing to grow beyond its focus on patient welfare. She was also prepared to use her own influence and position to gain advantage and benefit for the Society and its work.

The duchess was lucky to be supported by some able colleagues. It was common practice, for technical and administrative reasons, for organisations with the Society's structure to appoint a small number of trustees to hold the organisations land and other assets. Douglas Macmillan had persuaded his nephew Harold, a company director in the printing industry, to take on this role in 1957. He was later joined by Sir Richard Manktelow, formerly Deputy Secretary at the Ministry of Agriculture, Fisheries & Food and Douglas Macmillan's boss, and by Howard Challis, a city banker.

The Society's council, elected by the Society's members, also included men and women who could give good and reliable advice and direction. There was Sir Charles Davis, another of Macmillan's old colleagues from the civil service, who later became vice chairman with oversight of the Society's administration; there was Sir Alfred Broughton, a medical practitioner and Member of Parliament; and Sir William Geddis, businessman and Lord Mayor of Belfast. Moreover, many members of the Society's council, elected by the wider membership to represent local interests, also brought valuable skills and experience to the Society's deliberations. One was a city alderman, one managed a private nursing home, there were social workers, accountants and several doctors. Discussions at the full council could be animated affairs, with differing opinions and strongly held views being freely and energetically put across.

One of the first problems the duchess had to face was the expiry of the leases of the Society's offices in Victoria Street, which had by now expanded from number 47 to the adjoining number 45. Finding an alternative was not easy and the search took two years. The duchess had encouraged the philanthropist Michael (later Sir Michael) Sobell to accept the presidency of the Society after Macmillan's resignation. Sobell generously offered to donate to the Society the sum of nearly £60,000 for the purchase of a new head office. Characteristically, Sobell made this gift on the condition that it remained anonymous and that he received no public acknowledgement. This allowed the Society to acquire and refurbish 30 Dorset Square in Marylebone.

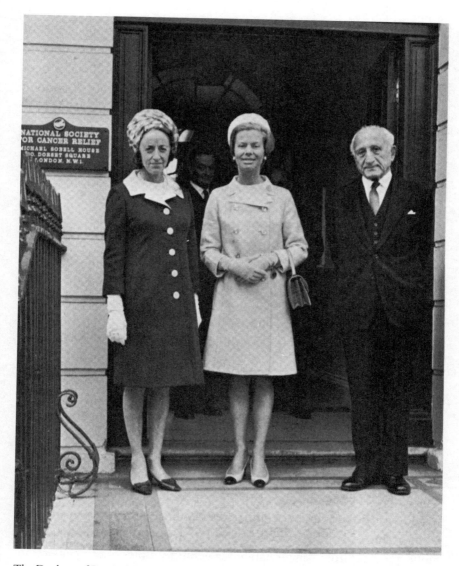

The Duchess of Roxburghe, the Duchess of Kent and Michael Sobell on the steps of the Society's new offices at 30 Dorset Square on 24 April 1967.

The building is an impressive Georgian town house, built as part of the Portman Estate. The staff at Victoria moved to their new office in July 1966. Sobell's gift included new furniture, carpets and equipment for the office, causing some bemusement, and even embarrassment, among the staff who were only used to second-hand.[1] At the beginning there was insufficient space to accommodate the staff of the welfare team and they remained in their old wartime office in Cheam. Later, planning permission was granted for the whole of the Dorset Square building to be used for offices and, after more than twenty years, the welfare team was reunited with the rest of the head office.

The second major achievement of this time was the agreement of the Duchess of Kent to become the Society's royal patron. The duchess, formerly Katharine Worsley, had been approached not long after her marriage in 1961 to the Duke of Kent and asked whether she would accept the position; but she was not ready to take on such a commitment. She did, however, agree to consider the offer again at a later time. The proposal was put a second time to the duchess, this time by the Duchess of Roxburghe in 1965, and in the following year she agreed to it. This was the beginning of an association between the Society and Katharine Kent, as she later preferred to be known, that would last for thirty-six years. She would give the Society a personal commitment and passion that far exceeded any hopes or expectations. She regularly attended the Society's Annual Meetings, often opening or closing the event with her own passionate words expressed from the heart. She opened buildings, met with doctors and nurses and encouraged them in their work. She would visit patients and talk with their families, offering sympathy and comfort. In return, the duchess received from the Society's members and supporters, and from cancer patients, a genuine and everlasting affection.

The biggest challenge that dominated the Society for the next ten years or so was how it could fulfil its commitment to provide nursing homes for people with cancer, and in particular for people whose cancer was incurable. The need for much better care of the terminally ill was beyond any doubt, or at least it was to people who had some direct experience of the care that was available. The Society's experience of setting up homes had been a pretty dismal one and one of the first initiatives of the new chairman was to improve the Society's relations with the Marie Curie Memorial Foundation, which had already opened a number of homes for cancer patients.

The Foundation had been founded in 1948 when the Marie Curie Hospital in Hampstead was absorbed by the National Health Service. A number of people associated with the hospital wanted to keep alive the memory of Marie Curie and so they started a charity in her name dedicated to relieving the sufferings of cancer patients. The first Marie Curie Home was opened in Scotland in 1952, and a further nine followed in all parts of the United Kingdom. Douglas Macmillan had been suspicious of this new charity, doubtless thinking that his own Society was already there to help people with cancer and that a new organisation was not needed.[2] His hostility was not helped by conflict over the use of the word 'relief' in fund-raising literature, and concern that the Foundation was in direct competition with the Society for funds. Indeed, the Society under Macmillan's lead had even declined to be referred to in the Foundation's literature, in case this might appear as some sort of endorsement from the Society.

It was clear to the Duchess of Roxburghe that some sensible accommodation between the two charities would be beneficial to all. She proposed, during the discussions that led to the closure of Helstonleigh, that the Society should concentrate on cancer relief, by which she meant patient welfare, and the Foundation should concentrate on operating nursing homes. As a part of this rapprochement, the Society offered to transfer Helstonleigh to the Foundation as a fully operating home.[3] While the Foundation was not prepared to restrict its work to operating nursing homes – it also funded nurse visitors – the discussions between the two organisations did produce an improvement in relations.

In early 1966, some supporters of the Society in Brighton, on the Sussex coast, were working independently on their own project to establish a nursing home for cancer patients. A local benefactor had offered a rent-free lease on a large house which could be converted into a nursing home for about twenty patients. A sum of money was available for the costs of conversion, but to make the project viable financial support was needed, at least in the short term, for operating costs. Some funding was assured from the National Assistance Board for the support of poor patients, and the Marie Curie Memorial

Foundation had promised help, but there was still a gap. The National Health Service at this time did not make funds available for care in non-NHS establishments.

Lord Cohen of Brighton, a local entrepreneur and politician, and Brighton doctor Jan de Winter, a specialist in cancer prevention, were leading the initiative. They envisaged that the home would be run by a management committee, separate from the Society's own Brighton committee. The Society was very positive about the project, and agreed to contribute £5,000 towards the first year's operating costs with the indication that regular support would be a possibility. This pledge was worth about one-third of annual operating costs, so it was quite instrumental in making the project financially viable. The society's treasurer, Dudley Chalk, joined the nursing home's management committee.

The nursing home, named Copper Cliff, became registered as a charity in its own right, and it welcomed its first patients in the spring of 1967. The Society was proud of its investment and received, through Chalk, regular reports on the progress of Copper Cliff. However, an annual grant towards the nursing home's general running costs did not really sit comfortably with the Society's focus on patient welfare, and in particular on relief to needy patients individually. As an alternative funding proposal, the Society pledged that it would set aside a sum each year from which the nursing home fees of those in most financial need would be met. The Society expected that patients who could afford it would make some financial contribution to their care. This, of course, had always been the position for patients cared for in private nursing or convalescent homes.

The Society's approach was understandable. It had limited funds available for its charitable work and its tradition had been to help the poor. In many ways, the Society was a charity working for the relief of the poor as much as for the relief of people with cancer. The Society saw an unwelcome precedent in making grants towards nursing home operating costs not linked to the financial means of its patients. There were many nursing homes, most of them in the private sector, but some in the charitable sector, which could care for cancer patients and could therefore apply for a block grant from the Society. The Society

did not want to be inundated with such requests. It much preferred
to support nursing homes within the context of its patient welfare
programme and its financial help for the needy. At the same time, the
Society fully understood that its own Brighton committee had led
fund-raising appeals for Copper Cliff and that it would no doubt do
so in the future. The income from local fund-raising for the Society
in Brighton and in the surrounding area of Sussex would, the Society
predicted, be reduced by the existence of Copper Cliff. However, the
Society was sanguine about this prospect, or at least it accepted that it
was inevitable.

At the same time as the opening of Copper Cliff, another home
for people with cancer was receiving its first patients. This was
St Christopher's Hospice, founded by Dr (later Dame) Cicely Saunders,
in Sydenham in south-east London. It was the first hospice to be
established in recent times, and a model for hundreds that would follow
in Britain and overseas.

In 1968 St Christopher's Hospice applied to the Society for
financial support and a sum of £10,000 was agreed, to be allocated
for patients in need along the same lines as the funding provided
for Copper Cliff. This grant was repeated, but within the Society
there was grumbling that the operating costs of the hospice were
twice as high as those at Copper Cliff and almost double those of
the Marie Curie Homes. There were even comments that the care
at St Christopher's was 'lavish'. Many members of the Society's local
committees thought that the priority for the Society should be to
help poor patients at home and not to support hospices at all. At
the same time, the Society's executive received reports that someone
at St Christopher's had accused the Society of being mean. Several
representatives from the Society visited St Christopher's Hospice to
see, at firsthand, the care given to patients, and they returned with
a much clearer understanding of the work of Dr Saunders and her
colleagues. They reported that the standard of care given to patients
'was incomparably higher', that the hospice's work 'went far beyond
that of the normal terminal care home', and that 'nothing which
helped to relieve the distress of sufferers' in the last few weeks of life
could be described as 'extravagant'. They also foresaw, significantly,

that 'other terminal care homes ... envisaged or under construction would model themselves on St Christopher's'.[4]

This was a welcome recognition of the ground-breaking importance of the work begun by Dr Saunders. Nevertheless, the Society still confirmed its policy of only giving financial support to patients in those nursing homes, or hospices, which demanded of patients who could afford it some contribution towards the costs of their care. This did not fulfil Douglas Macmillan's dream for care in homes to be given 'freely or at low cost', but the Society did not have the financial means – and huge they would have to have been to bring about the founder's dream.

At the same time, the reliance on other charities to fulfil Douglas Macmillan's vision to see 'a chain of homes for cancer patients throughout the land' would have been unduly passive and timid to say the least. After all, with income in 1967 of close to £400,000, free reserves of a similar amount, a UK-wide network of committees and supporters, and a growing status in the field, the Society was in a position to give some leadership. Moreover, during the 1960s while the Society's income was growing, the number of applications for welfare support remained pretty constant, indicating that, at least on the existing criteria for payments, the Society had reached some sort of plateau. This was despite,

> all the efforts made to seek out cancer sufferers in need of help made by the Society's members and its Committees, by other voluntary organisations, by the social welfare departments of hospitals, doctors, consultants, the clergy and others ...[5]

The Society was increasingly successful and was getting too big for its quite limited range of activities, while at the same time, patients still had critical needs that were not being met. The Society reported that it 'heard constantly of people who had died of cancer at home and before they could obtain a bed in a hospital' and it had to admit that it 'had funds available for relief but inadequate outlets for their proper disposal, while on the other hand the need for terminal care homes was clear'.

The Society drew the obvious conclusion that it ought to use its funds to help set up new homes. The problem was how to do it. It set up its own study group to examine the need for nursing homes and to decide the location of new ones to be built.

The study group set about its work in October 1968 by consulting other charities, including the Marie Curie Memorial Foundation and also the Ministry of Health. By the following July the group had concluded that homes were needed, as the first priority, in southern Lancashire, the north Midlands and near the Yorkshire and Durham border. These were areas without Marie Curie Homes or alternative facilities. The chairman of the study group was chartered accountant Edward Buxton, a strong-willed and confident man[6] who was determined to break with the modest progress of the recent years. He was a member of the Society's council and also chairman of its North Staffordshire Committee. Another member of the group was a radiologist, Dr Derek Meredith-Brown, who practised in the same area. The Potteries, as the area was more commonly known, consisted of the towns of Stoke-on-Trent and Newcastle-under-Lyme and the surrounding mining areas. They were heavily industrial and the centre of the ceramics industry. The North Staffordshire Committee was eager to build and operate a home for cancer patients – indeed the idea had first been canvassed in 1962 because,

> It was ... clear that a number of patients with cancer ... were unable to cope and required help which could not be found in their own homes. ... Moreover, hospitals had neither the space nor staff to care for patients. ... Some patients with cancer faced a wait for a hospital bed which was longer than their life expectancy.[7]

Encouragingly, the North Staffordshire Committee, which had been founded by the Lord Mayor of Stoke at Frank Georgeson's suggestion, promised it would undertake to raise annually sufficient funds for the home's operating costs. What the committee needed was a major capital sum from the Society to build the home. The Society saw great merit in the proposal; it could be instrumental in establishing a new home for cancer patients in an area of particular need – north Staffordshire can be described as the north Midlands – but without taking responsibility for day-to-day management or the yearly running costs. The only condition that the Society wanted to apply to its financial contribution was that the new home be named the Douglas Macmillan Home after the Society's founder. This was at the instigation of Dudley Chalk, who had suggested that an appropriate memorial to Douglas Macmillan would be the foundation of homes bearing his name. The naming proposal was agreed to and a capital grant of £50,000 was approved.

At almost the same time, the Society received from the Bishop of Manchester an appeal for support for a project to build a home for the terminally ill in Manchester. Dr Eric Easson, a member of the Society's council who was also the director of the Radiotherapy Centre at the Christie Hospital, strongly supported the project, as did the Society's Manchester Committee. Easson argued that the Marie Curie Home in Liverpool was too far away to cater for people from the Manchester conurbation as well and that the Society's support for the initiative at that early stage would be critical to its success. The Society agreed to make a contribution to equal that promised to the north Staffordshire project. The Society wanted the Manchester home also to be named after Douglas Macmillan, but the name St Ann's Hospice had already been settled upon.

The financial obligation of £100,000 for the two new hospices was a very large one for the Society. Indeed, it was the largest commitment of funds it had ever made (although it represented no more than the Society's surplus of income over expenditure for the previous year). There were some voices of dissent. One Society member from the Brierley Hill Committee expressed concern that such a large grant would be made to Manchester when the Society's Manchester Committee had only raised £300 for the Society in the previous year. But this was a parochial view. Others stressed that the Society had to help where the need was greatest, without regard to a locality's fund-raising achievements. This was an important point of principle.

In due course, St Ann's Hospice in Cheadle, to the south of Manchester, received its first patients on 17 May 1971. The opening of the Douglas Macmillan Home at Barlaston, a suburb of Stoke, took place on 2 January 1973.[8] Not surprisingly, once the word got round

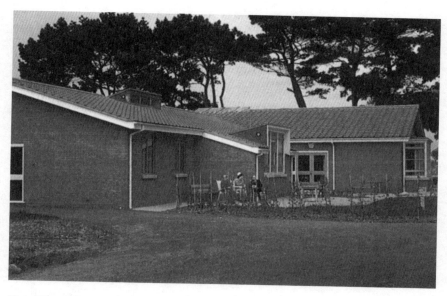

New Macmillan unit at Christchurch.

that the Society would make capital sums available for new hospice development, the number of requests began to grow. St Luke's Nursing Home in Sheffield was one of the first, and the Society made a grant to cover the purchase of the twenty-five beds that the hospice would need; a sum of £10,000 was also given towards the construction of the St Barnabas Hospice in Worthing.

The scheme, however, that was of particular interest to the Society was a proposal put forward by the National Health Service, or rather by its Bournemouth and East Dorset Hospital Management Committee. This was for the construction of a home on the site of the NHS Christchurch Hospital with, significantly, the NHS undertaking to meet all of the new hospice's operating costs. The force behind the project was Dr Ronald Fisher, a consultant anaesthetist with a strong interest in pain control.[9] The attraction for the Society was obvious. The Society could make its capital grant in the knowledge that there would be no recurrent requests for assistance with operating costs and that its local committee would not need to become a perpetual fund-raising machine for the new service. The local committee, on the contrary, could continue to raise funds for the welfare work of the Society.

The Society readily pledged £35,000 towards the construction of the building, conditional upon the new home taking the name of Douglas Macmillan. Although the Hospital Management Committee had a policy of not naming buildings after people, and was at first reluctant to cede to the Society's request, the Society made it clear that the condition was not negotiable and the deal was done.

It was clear to the Society that it could play an important, and sometimes pivotal, role in the development of homes for people with cancer by using the Fisher model. Douglas Macmillan's dream could, after all, become a reality. It was also clear that the Society would have to grow if it was to have income necessary to make so many of these large capital grants available for new hospice building. The new homes had to be paid for in addition to the programme of welfare payments, and not at their expense.

The year 1971 marked the 60th anniversary of William Macmillan's death and Douglas Macmillan's resolve to establish the Society, and this was a major opportunity to begin a fund-raising appeal for money to build the much-needed homes for cancer patients. It was called the Lillian Board Cancer Clinic Appeal. Lillian Board, from Manchester, had been a hero of British athletics. She had won a silver medal at the 1968 Olympics and two gold medals at the European championships the following year. She was attractive, engaging and much loved, and great things were expected of her in the Olympic Games of 1972. Tragically, in 1970 she was diagnosed with advanced cancer of the bowel. In desperation Board's family took her for treatment to a controversial cancer clinic in Bavaria run by Dr Josef Issels, but she died on Boxing Day that year. She was just 22. The appeal was the idea of Jeffrey Archer[10] and his fund-raising company Arrow Enterprises, which had been recommended to the Society by Michael Sobell. The appeal was criticised for coming too soon after the athlete's death, but nevertheless it was launched by the Duchess of Roxburghe on 6 April 1971 with the full support of Lillian Board's family. The duchess said of Lillian that she was, 'Not only a great and beloved athlete, but a wonderful person. Her death will not have passed without purpose'. It was the biggest fund-raising project ever embarked upon by the Society, with a target of £1 million. It was planned to use the fund

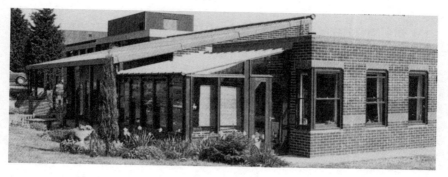

The new home for cancer patients at Oxford.

to build as many new homes for cancer patients as the income would allow.

One of the first donations to be associated with the Lillian Board Appeal was from the Society's president, Sir Michael Sobell. Sobell offered £100,000 (later increased to £138,000) to finance a home for cancer patients in southern England. The Society was grateful indeed for such support and generosity and the preferred location for the building came to be Oxford. Just as in the project at Christchurch, a local NHS hospital, in this case the Churchill Hospital, was keen to have the new building on site. The Society did not have a fund-raising committee in Oxford and it needed a commitment from the NHS to cover the new home's operating costs. This was not readily forthcoming and there was much argument inside the NHS about whether the responsibility should be borne by the Regional Hospital Board, the United Oxford Hospitals Management Committee or the Department of Health and Social Security. Indeed, at one point Sobell became understandably impatient with the delay, and there was even worry that Sobell's offer might be withdrawn altogether. Happily, the matter was resolved.

Meanwhile, the task of assessing the need for facilities for cancer patients had been passed to the British Cancer Council, a discussion forum consisting of representatives from the major cancer charities and government departments. It was not easy work because of the paucity of relevant statistics maintained by the National Health Service or within the Ministry of Health. In due course, the council concluded that the need was greatest in Nottingham, the Portsmouth and Southampton conurbation, in Glasgow and on the western fringes of Greater London, but identifying the place of need was not the biggest problem. The Society had learned enough to know that new homes for cancer patients, or continuing care homes as they were being called, could not be conjured into existence. Building projects required skilled and effective management that cut across architecture and design, construction, cost controls, planning and finance. Services for patients needed direction and practical, professional supervision. It was not at all clear that the Society had this level and spread of expertise. Most importantly, successful projects came with the demanding burden of yearly operating costs. The Society concluded that if its programme of construction was to continue in a logical and needs-driven way, it needed the support and cooperation of the Department of Health and Social Security. In effect this meant that, for the future, the approval of the Regional Hospital Board of the NHS would be an essential prerequisite for the Society's commitment to any project.

The Society had clearly established its preferred way of operating. It would make grants but leave it to others to run the services. This was unusual for a fund-raising charity. Most grant-giving charities had endowed funds specifically for this purpose. As a result, the Society began to receive many requests for help from other charities endeavouring to help people with cancer. The Society helped when it could, but mostly funding was limited.

The Society did take on the responsibility of funding a small number of other charities on a permanent basis. The first was a small charity called the British Colostomy Association. The number of patients suffering with cancers of the bowel had steadily increased, and the standard treatment was surgical removal of the diseased section of bowel. Often patients were left with a temporary or permanent colostomy. This very specialised charity offered much-needed support and advice to patients who were about to undergo, or who had undergone, this particularly drastic surgical procedure with its very unpleasant outcome.

The Colostomy Welfare Group, as it was then called, first approached the Society in 1970, and requested a grant of £5,000 to cover the bulk of its operating costs. The group reported that it found fund-raising for the cause extremely difficult. The Society, with strong encouragement from trustee Manktelow, agreed the request for support and continued to do so on a yearly basis. A similar request for support came in 1976 from the National Association of Laryngectomee Clubs. Cancer of the larynx or voice box, usually caused by smoking, was also becoming more common. The surgical removal of the larynx left patients unable to speak and having to breathe through an opening into the windpipe in the neck. Local laryngectomee clubs provided for patients similar support to that provided by the Colostomy Association to its patients. The third charity to join this group was the Breast Care and Mastectomy Association[11] in 1981, and the last, in 1987, was Cancerlink, an umbrella group supporting cancer self-help groups. These four charities became known as 'associated charities', using a term borrowed from the commercial world.

The Society's support for these charities served several purposes. Most importantly it enabled the Society to provide some of those patient information and support services that had been a part of Douglas Macmillan's hope for the future. It is certainly true that the survival of one or more of these charities would have been most unlikely without the Society's continuous support. The Society considered whether it should just take over all the affairs of the four, and absorb them, but it preferred, on balance, to maintain an arm's length relationship. This was more in keeping with the Society's policy of providing the funds to others who would give the service. In return for financial support, the 'associated charities' had to undertake not to raise funds in competition with the Society's own fund-raising, and they had to acknowledge the Society's support.

In the longer term, the 'associated charities' did begin to eat more and more of the Society's resources, and the Society became less comfortable with their total dependence. In due course they were encouraged to go it alone. The Breast Care and Mastectomy Association became fully self-supporting fifteen years after it first received the Society's funds, the British Colostomy Association continued to receive funding until 2005 and Cancerlink was ultimately absorbed by the Society altogether in 2001.

★★★

When the Duchess of Roxburghe became chairman of the Society in 1963, it had an income of a little more than £300,000 (about £3.9 million today), rising to nearly £600,000 in 1970. By the end of 1972, and twenty months after the launch of the Lillian Board Appeal, annual income had exceeded £1 million for the first time. Ten years later and income had grown to nearly £2.7 million (about £5.9 million today), although inflation made this increase more apparent than real. Nevertheless, the growth was steady and continuous.

This growth of income came about, in part, as a result of the Society's diversification into nursing homes and other services and the wider public interest and support that accompanied them. But fund-raising was still a huge challenge that had to be met every year. The duchess's role was a key element in the success as she worked both to raise the Society's profile and to encourage the efforts of others.

Horse racing was a Roxburghe passion and she made a link between the Society and the turf which survived for the remainder of the century. She helped to instigate a National Cancer Day for the benefit of the Society, the Marie Curie Memorial Foundation and the British Empire Cancer Campaign during the Ascot race meeting in 1967. It was a keen part of her philosophy that the cancer charities should work together. The event raised nearly £28,000 for each charity. It was repeated the following year and evolved into several events.

Eventually, under the sponsorship of the Hambro family, the loose organisation became the Joint Cancer Charities Council and each year organised the prestigious Businessman of the Year Award Luncheon. The duchess was instrumental in securing the support of Timeform, the racing publications company, with events at race meetings at Doncaster and York. Timeform became a long-term supporter of the Society.

The duchess also persuaded many of her friends to support the Society, and new networks of supporters were created. Sobell, Hambro, Rollo, Halifax and Tennant were all names that became associated with the Society through the Roxburghe connection. But the duchess was not solely interested in recruiting supporters from high society. She was just as assiduous at paying attention to the Society's small and local committees of volunteers, and during her time the number of committees rapidly grew. She travelled the United Kingdom widely,

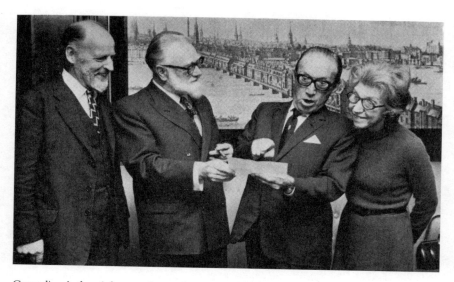

Comedian Arthur Askey receives a cheque on behalf of the Society from Philip Bull of Timeform. Jeremy Shaw and Irene Askey look on.

meeting with local supporters and encouraging them in their work for the Society.

The duchess's efforts were well supported and complemented by others. A Greater London Committee was formed in 1971 under the chairmanship of Lord Irwin (later the Earl of Halifax) and it organised a spate of events including a preview at Christies, and gala showings of the film *The Godfather* one year, followed by *Paper Moon* the next. The Society's committee in Glasgow was given the film premiere of *Murder on the Orient Express*. Also in Scotland, the Pineapple ProCelAm Golf Tournament was the biggest of its kind ever organised for charity. Meanwhile, the Society had appointed a new appeals secretary to take on responsibility for fund-raising.[12] This was Hugh Shaw, a retired commander from the Fleet Air Arm. Shaw was a dynamic and hardworking man. He was always looking out for new ideas to raise money and he had an ability to get people to do things.[13] Notable events to raise money included a concert by pianist Moura Lympany in the presence of the Prince of Wales at St James's Palace; a boxing evening at the Café Royal featuring a bout between Henry Cooper and his brother George; and a 'Ski-do' held on the slopes of the dry ski run at Lord's cricket ground with competing teams from the Houses of

Parliament, Oxford, Cambridge, Fleet Street, the City, the Army and the Navy. The Duke of Kent captained the team from the Army.

It was an indication of the growing status of the Society that it could call on people at all levels and from all walks of life to support its fund-raising events. None, though, could have been more distinguished than the legendary crooner from America, Bing Crosby, who appeared at the London Palladium in June 1976 to mark his 50th anniversary in show business. A friend of the Society's London organiser, Mary Henderson, Crosby donated his entire fee to charity, one-half of it going to the Society. Joan Bebbington, Relief Secretary at the time, recalled Crosby walking to the Society's offices in Dorset Square on the morning of the first concert and meeting informally the Society's staff. Few people can include chatting to one of the world's most famous entertainers as part of their day's work.

Probably the most ambitious event, or rather non-event, from the period was the Queen Elizabeth II Charity Cruise. The idea was Shaw's, but the duchess pursued it with enthusiasm. In 1968 the new Cunard liner, known to everyone as the *QE2*, was 'booked' by the Society for its first ever passenger voyage. It was due to sail from Southampton on 23 December and return four days later. This was a dress rehearsal for the ship's maiden voyage to New York. A great deal of work was essential to organise the event, and there was insufficient time available to sell all of the passages. Nevertheless, the level of disappointment can only be imagined when Cunard cancelled the trip on 8 December because of the ship's engine problems. The Society's costs were covered by insurance and the aborted event still brought the Society about £20,000 in donations. However, a remarkable and unique fund-raising event was lost.

Of course, a major proportion of the Society's income came not from grand events but from the continuing enthusiasm and activity of the Society's local committees. The number grew from 177 in 1964 to 296 in 1972. Five years later there were 437 committees. In 1976 the committees raised a total of £498,572 (about £2.3 million today), about 30 per cent of the Society's total income. Another 30 per cent came from legacies to the Society, with special events contributing about 12 per cent. Given that the local committees were comprised entirely of volunteers, many of them retired or with other commitments, some of their successes were outstanding. Several committees raised more than £5,000. Star performers were the Southend Committee which raised £7,250; Hastings which raised £7,816, and Newport and Gwent which each raised £6,000. But the truly remarkable committees were Glasgow and Edinburgh, which raised £12,500 (about £56,000 today) and £18,782 respectively. By now, the Society had thirteen regional organisers (eleven remunerated), who supported committees and developed new ones, and regional offices had been opened in Liverpool and Birmingham. The Society's national base was growing wider and deeper.

The growth of the Society in the duchess's first few years had been significant. The Society had branched out from patient welfare grants to nursing home or hospice construction, and its income was expanding to finance this new endeavour. It was becoming a complex business operation and needed professional management. On the other hand, the structure of the Society had not changed in response to all this growth. It was, instead, much as Douglas Macmillan had left it. It was still led and managed, for the most part, by volunteers. The salaried staff, headed by general secretary Gordon Tredwell, a retired squadron leader and district commissioner from Rhodesia, were essential for the smooth day-to-day workings of the organisation. Often, though, they were administrators and there to support voluntary executives.

There was a growing concern of the duchess and her colleagues that this structure would no longer do, and that it would become increasingly ineffective as the Society continued to get bigger and as it attempted to do more. Sir Charles Davis, who in 1972 became a vice chairman with responsibility for administration and establishment, recommended that a review of the Society's 'structure, organisation, methods and accommodation' be undertaken, and that an external consultant be recruited to assist with this review. Davis said that the 'object was to ensure that the Society was geared for the growth ... confidently expected in the next few years, and to identify and cure any major problems which might adversely affect it'.

The review would be undertaken by Davis's sub-committee comprising of Sir Richard Manktelow, treasurer Stanley and the general secretary. The name of Major Henry Garnett was suggested as someone who might be the consultant to assist with the task. He came highly recommended by Stanley, who had known him for many years, and it was agreed that the review would begin in the autumn of 1972.

By the time the executive committee of the Society met on 30 November 1972, vice chairman Davis was able to circulate a paper with his sub-committee's recommendations. They were radical, and represented a step change in the way the organisation was managed. Davis proposed that a new salaried post of deputy chairman and chief executive be created. The post-holder would be responsible for preparing short- and long-terms plans for the Society, for budgets and budgetary control, and for the implementation of plans and policies. Importantly, the post-holder would chair meetings of the executive. For the first time in the Society's history, a salaried official would take over the driving seat.

Davis then went further and recommended that Henry Garnett be appointed to the position. The proposals met with disagreement. Strong opposition to the recommendations came particularly from many of the local committee representatives. They complained of the costs of employing an additional senior member of staff, and especially one who would likely cost rather more than the others. They expressed concern that a new officer would be superimposed on the existing staff and structures, and they aired their reservations about Garnett who had no experience of medicine or health care. Moreover, according to one observer,[14] the case for change was not helped by Davis and his colleagues giving the appearance of trying to railroad other members of the executive and council. In any event, the stage was set for confrontation at the special general meeting of members, which had to be held in order to agree to the changes that would be required.

The special meeting was held on 6 February 1973 in the meeting hall of the Royal Commonwealth Society in London. It was a very poorly attended meeting with just thirty members of the Society present.[15] This may have been a reflection on the constitutionally sufficient but nevertheless short notice given for the meeting, or that generally most members of the Society did not regard the issue as quite so fundamental.

Opponents of the changes spoke of their 'bitter resentment', demanded more information about the proposals to take back to their

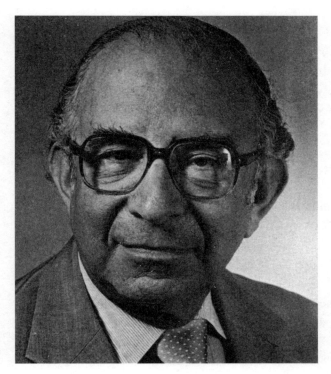

Charles Davis.

committees and predicted an exodus of members if the meeting passed the resolution in front of it. By contrast, the treasurer said that he had become increasingly convinced that the management of the Society had to be modernised. He was backed strongly by Jocelyn Hambro, recently retired as chairman of Hambros Bank, who argued that running a charity was the same as running a business, with large sums of money held in trust. For her part, the duchess let it be known that she would find it difficult to continue as chairman if the proposals were thrown out. The officers won the day, with a vote of 17 in favour of the changes and 10 against. This was a great triumph for the modernisers and for those who were looking to the future. It would push the Society many rungs up the ladder.

The Duchess of Roxburghe continued as the Society's chairman for another ten years, working closely with Garnett. As Mrs Jocelyn Hambro from 1976, she continued to play her part with diligence and aplomb, and according to observers she always had 'a buzz about her'.[16]

Unfortunately, and as so often happened to those associated with the Society's story, in 1979 she was diagnosed with cancer. Despite the best of treatments available in Britain and the United States of America, she was given just one year to live. In fact, she proved the doctors wrong and outlived their expectations, but she died of the illness in 1983.

Notes & References

1. Interview with Joan Bebbington, 6 June 2005.
2. To some extent Macmillan may have been right. The Marie Curie Memorial Foundation was set up to give practical help to people with cancer after their discharge from hospital, and so it incorporated welfare grants and nursing care, as well as nursing homes. However, the Foundation's pilot, the distinguished London cancer surgeon Ronald Raven, would doubtless have found it very difficult to work within the limits of the Society. Indeed, the Foundation had established its network of cancer homes, Marie Curie centres, before the Society had any success in the field.
3. After some initial interest, the Foundation decided not to take it on, probably because of the same financial reasoning that had led to the Society deciding to close the home.
4. Reported in minutes of the Society's executive committee meeting of 17 March 1970.
5. Annual report of the Society for 1969.
6. Ibid., Bebbington.
7. *Douglas Macmillan Hospice: The first Twenty-five Years*, edited by Myrtle Summerly, published by Douglas Macmillan Hospice, 1997.
8. The progress of the project was delayed because of planning and other problems.
9. Fisher was an important figure in the development of palliative care services in the UK and overseas. He was a pioneer of Macmillan nursing and of hospice day care services. He died in 2007 aged 90.
10. At the time, Archer was Member of Parliament for Louth and a rising star of the Conservative Party. He has since become Lord Archer of Weston-super-Mare, and was infamously sent to prison for perjury in 2001.
11. Now called Breast Cancer Care.

12. Georgeson had left the Society in 1963.

13. Ibid., Bebbington. Shaw died tragically from a heart attack in 1977.

14. Ibid., Bebbington, conversation with author on 6 June 2005.

15. Annual General Meetings usually attracted more than 100 members. With more than 7,000 members, the attendance on this occasion was less than 0.5 per cent.

16. *From JOH*, by Andrew St George, 1992, unpublished.

10

The Major Takes Over

Henry Claud Lyon Garnett was born in October 1913, so he was just under 60 years of age when he took up his post of deputy chairman and chief executive of the Society. Educated at Eton and Sandhurst, he had served as an officer in the Royal Horse Guards, both before and during the Second World War, retiring with the rank of major. Back in civilian life, Garnett joined Gillette, the American shaving products company. After postings in the United States and Australia he became chairman of Gillette's UK subsidiary, and then, based in France, chairman of Gillette's European operation. He was awarded the CBE when Gillette UK won the Queen's Award for Industry and, in 1963, Garnett was responsible for initiating the cricket tournament called the Gillette Cup. Garnett came to the Society as a very senior executive with an impressive career in business and management behind him. He also came with a little experience of charity work. He had played a leading role starting new boys' clubs in Middlesex, and he had been a member of the council of the British Heart Foundation.[1] Garnett was a very tall,[2] smart and distinguished-looking man, who commanded respect

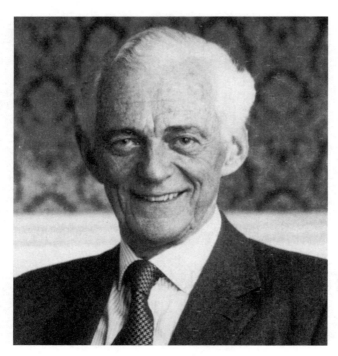

Henry Garnett.

and much affection from those who worked with him. He was a canny operator and a clever negotiator with a businessman's head for seizing advantage and opportunity. His contribution to the work of the Society would be second only to that of Douglas Macmillan himself.

At the beginning, the controversy over Garnett's appointment rumbled on until the Society's Annual Meeting held in June 1973. There, a few malcontents tried to have the whole matter reconsidered, but they could muster only nine votes out of the 130 or more members present. And in any event, Garnett began to show his worth very quickly. He introduced proper yearly budgeting, and he improved accounting and reporting systems to provide the Society with more effective management controls. Within a few months, general secretary Tredwell decided to retire, and this allowed Garnett to go ahead with a major restructuring of the office and its staffing. Responsibility for much of the contact and liaison with the local committees was transferred from head office to the network of regional organisers, and suppliers of stationery and other goods were made to deal directly with committees rather than through a head office intermediary. This allowed for more streamlined working and a reduction of head office administrative staff from twelve to eight.

Coupled with this, Garnett introduced a computerised accounting system for patient welfare payments which allowed the number of people employed in the relief team to fall from eleven to four. Altogether, Garnett cut the head office staff complement by one-third. The savings he made were used, in part, to increase the number of staff in fund-raising based outside London, and to establish more regional offices. Garnett also set about improving some rates of pay and working conditions for the remaining staff in order to make the Society more competitive in the jobs market. One of the Society's problems had been difficulty in recruiting and retaining good-quality staff, with an inevitable impact on organisational performance. Garnett's tight control over head office staff levels was not a short-term policy. With some ups and downs, in 1980, after several years of growth and development, still only twenty-four people were employed at the head office.

The other pressing problem for the new chief executive had been the shortage of space at the Dorset Square office, coupled with the dislocation to efficient working caused by the welfare team still operating from Cheam. Applications for welfare payments to patients were considered and approved by case officers based at Cheam, but they then had to be referred to the Dorset Square office for authorisation and for the cheques to be drawn. This inevitably meant that staff had to travel regularly between the two offices and there was the risk of delay to patients receiving their grants. The Society had gone so far as to agree in principle that a search be conducted for alternative premises, big enough to accommodate the Dorset Square and the Cheam staff, although nothing suitable was found. However, Garnett's reduction of head office staff levels and the elimination of much storage requirement, meant that there was now enough space for the Cheam staff at last to be moved to Dorset Square and re-integrated with the Society's other head office functions. Efficiency could be improved and a financial saving made on the Cheam office rental. The process of transfer was not without difficulty and the computerised payments system had early teething problems. But still, the Duchess of Roxburghe was able to report at the Annual Meeting held in June 1974 that the move was complete, and a start had been made in the head office to catch up with the backlog of work caused by the poor systems and inadequate management of recent years.

Garnett's biggest task of his early years was to bring greater energy and direction to the Society's programme of nursing home building and construction. Indeed, the duchess had used the apparent lethargy of the programme as one of her arguments for Garnett's appointment. She was sad that at the beginning of 1973, two years after the launch of the appeal, 'not a single Lillian Board Memorial Clinic had yet been started'.

This may not have been a fair comment because major construction projects do take some time to be planned, executed and completed. But it was surely true that the Society's record was poor compared with that of the Marie Curie Memorial Foundation which had established ten new homes in a little more than twenty years and which, under the influence of the extremely successful surgeon Ronald Raven, was increasingly taking a leading role in cancer care and rehabilitation. Within months, Garnett had embarked upon a series of visits to potential nursing home locations throughout England, Scotland and Wales, meeting local NHS health boards and exploring the possibility of collaboration. Treasurer Stanley and vice chairman Davis had encouraged him to put together a five-year plan for new home construction, with the ambitious target of starting two new projects each year. Apart from the Oxford project, which had already been approved, developments had been proposed for Portsmouth or Southampton, Nottingham, Northampton and Peterborough. Garnett was also encouraged to plan a new fund-raising drive to support this major growth of the building programme.[3]

Garnett's approach to his discussions with the NHS boards was based on Fisher's successful collaborative project at the Christchurch Hospital. The regional hospital board of the NHS had to provide, at no cost to the Society, a site for the building either at an existing hospital or adjacent to it. The Society would then pay for the capital cost of the new building, or it would share the cost with a local fund-raising group, but thereafter the service would have to be managed by the hospital board, which would also take responsibility for all future operating costs. The Society also needed to approve the hospital board's operational plans for the unit, and to be represented on any project or planning committee. This approach was quite different from that of the Marie Curie Memorial Foundation, and from the voluntary associations which had established Copper Cliff, St Christopher's Hospice and the other homes for cancer patients. These other charities had been established to be the direct operators of inpatient care services. The Society, probably still conscious of the failure of Helstonleigh, was determined instead to be a developer of, or a catalyst for, new inpatient services. It did not want to be an operator of them too.

The work of Cicely Saunders at St Christopher's Hospice had a huge impact on the care of the dying, and in particular of those dying from cancer. The model of St Christopher's was soon copied widely, not only in Britain but in other countries too, earning Saunders the unofficial title of 'Founder of the Modern Hospice Movement', and later the highest official honours of Dame of the British Empire and the Order of Merit.[4] A part of the hospice thesis was that the hospitals of the NHS, and those in the private sector for that matter, were wholly absorbed in attempts to cure patients of their cancers, often irrespective of whether or not cure was possible. Terminal illness was regarded as a medical or surgical failure, and it attracted few of the NHS's scarce resources. Dying patients were cared for in general hospital wards or sent home to die, often in great pain and distress. They were rarely given the intensive medical and nursing attention they needed, let alone any psychological and social support. The words 'I am afraid there is nothing more we can do' were a real part of everyday hospital life, as well as a caricature from weepy films at the cinema. It was no coincidence that all of the early hospice developments occurred in the voluntary sector, unbridled by the mainstream and the orthodoxy of those leading the National Health Service.

By the time of Garnett's arrival at the Society things were beginning to change. There was a growing number of people within the National Health Service who accepted that the NHS's commitment to provide care 'from the cradle to the grave' was seriously lacking at the mors mortis end of the spectrum. NHS hospitals at the time were still administered through the structure set up by health minister Bevan in 1947. The teaching hospitals were managed by boards of governors and

the others, the majority, by hospital management committees responsible
to regional hospital boards. Decision-making tended to be geared to the
needs of powerful consultants and a few other dominant or persuasive
people. This explains why the care of terminally ill patients was often
neglected – palliative medicine was not a recognised speciality then –
but also why it could be given much greater priority if it had a powerful
champion to argue its case. More and more people within the NHS,
often influenced by the work of St Christopher's, began to push for the
development of hospices as an integral part of the state system. Fisher
had been but the first of these, at Christchurch, and now Garnett was
able to make common cause with many others across the UK.

Between 1973 and 1979, no fewer than nine large-scale inpatient
units were completed for the NHS, and a further two were in hand.
These included the units at Christchurch and Oxford, which had been
planned a year earlier, and also units at Northampton, Southampton,
Northwood, Dundee, Aberdeen, Norwich and Nottingham. Cambridge
and Swansea would be completed in 1981. Most of these new centres
contained twenty or twenty-five inpatient beds for patients whose
illnesses were terminal. Patients might be admitted temporarily for
review and control of their symptoms or to give their carers at home
some respite, or for the very last stages of the illness. The large majority
of patients would have incurable cancer; a few would be suffering from
other terminal illnesses, such as motor neurone disease. The centres
aimed to provide all of the expert medical and nursing care for the
terminally ill that recent research and modern practice could offer, and
also the special care and attention for patients and families that had
been pioneered in the voluntary hospices. With their own facilities
for teaching and research, these units could replicate the work of St
Christopher's, and they could often attract staff of the highest calibre.
To give just one example, Dr Robert Twycross, a protégé of Cicely
Saunders and later an international expert in the palliative medicine,
became the consultant physician at the unit in Oxford.

In one aspect, the hospital units diverged from the pattern established
from St Christopher's. They shunned the word 'hospice' and used the
word 'house' instead. This was probably because of a feeling that the
word 'hospice' conjured up the wrong impression in the mind of

patient and family. It was still not generally acceptable to talk of death and dying. For many it remained a subject of taboo, with echoes of the words spoken by Lord Webb-Johnson in the House of Lords twenty years before. The word 'hospice' also had a religious connotation, perhaps with an implication that here the dying could be close to God. Although Cicely Saunders had readily used the word 'hospice' in 1967, it is interesting to record that in Sheffield, St Luke's Nursing Home was not renamed St Luke's Hospice until 1985, and that the Marie Curie Homes were not called hospices until even later.

It was for this sort of reason that the Society decided that its inpatient units 'should not be given names that directly associated them with the work of the society'. The word 'cancer' had to be avoided. At the time, even the Society's welfare payments to patients were sent via a third party, usually an almoner or social worker, so that the patient would not receive a cheque with the ominous words *National Society for* **Cancer Relief** written beneath the signatures. The Society instead decided that the buildings should be named after individuals associated in some way with their beginnings. The units at Oxford and Northwood were named after Michael Sobell, their benefactor; the units in Aberdeen and Dundee were called after the Duchess of Roxburghe; the Southampton unit became Countess Mountbatten House after the Society's late president;[5] in Northampton, Cynthia Spencer House was named after the Countess Spencer who had been president of the local appeal for funds.[6] Collectively, the centres built by the Society were called the 'continuing care units',[7] and they soon became known as '*Macmillan* continuing care units', in honour of the Society's founder.

The development of each new continuing care unit was a major undertaking. A brief had to be prepared detailing all the user requirements from the number of beds, cabinets and cupboards, to the location of the WCs, baths and treatment rooms. Most patients in the unit would be very ill, so it was important to get the unit's design aligned with the day-to-day operational needs from the very beginning. Architects would then draw up final plans which would, after consultation with quantity surveyors, be the basis of an invitation to builders to tender a price for the construction. Meanwhile, issues of town planning and building regulations had to be cleared. In these early schemes, the Society was the principal party in all the legal contracts, so the preparatory work was both exhaustive and detailed. It would have absorbed a great deal of time of the few senior staff at the Society. This was not sound business in Garnett's mind. He wanted a way of reducing this workload on the Society.

The Oxford Regional Hospital Board had, in the early 1960s, developed its own system of construction, encouraged by the programme of hospital building launched by Minister of Health, Enoch Powell.[8] The board had a big capital development programme and was concerned about the very long time it took between the initial stages of planning to completion. Several years was normal. Taking advantage of new building materials such as metals and plastics, standardised components, factory-built units and final assembly on site, the hospital board's architects developed what became known in building and construction as the Oxford Method. So long as structures and designs could be rationalised and made simple, the Oxford Method of systems building could produce results at very economic cost and in quick time. The continuing care unit at Oxford, in the grounds of Headington Hospital and the first built by this system, cost a little more than £200,000. It was followed by Cynthia Spencer House at the Manfield Hospital in Northampton, which cost £233,515. The Northampton project took just two years from preliminary brief to completion. Since the Society's projects were not subject to the growing bureaucracy of the Department of Health and Social Security, they could be completed without the delays that inevitably accompanied Whitehall interference.

Garnett saw the Oxford Method as the one to use for the Society's other continuing care units. Outside of the Oxford NHS area, the Oxford Method had been licensed to a company called C.E.D. Building Services. As well as managing health buildings construction projects for clients, the company could even operate the range of health care and ancillary services that a new building would need. The company was a Private Finance Initiative contractor some twenty years before that concept of public service procurement had supposedly been thought of. Garnett was quick to engage C.E.D. Building Services for the Society's projects, and at the beginning of 1974 the company was retained as the Society's construction programme consultants for all NHS developments.

The one disadvantage of the Oxford Method, and it was a big one, was that designs and materials that would provide suitable accommodation for acute hospital services, did not necessarily work so well for a home for the terminally ill. A part of the hospice concept was that the building could often be the patient's last home, and prefabricated, standardised building shells were not always easy to make homely. Nevertheless, the system allowed for a rapid growth of patient services over a short time vista. Each unit would admit on average 300 patients a year. So, by 1982, as a result of the Society's work constructing these units for the NHS, some 3,300 more people each year were receiving the special inpatient care they so much needed at the end of life, and which hitherto had just not been there. Dr Robert Dickson, medical director of Michael Sobell House in Northwood said:

> We're not trying to cure here, but to make life comfortable and death both painless and free of fear. Our failures are not those who eventually die – we know that in most cases that is inevitable – but those who die in pain.

The Society's plan was to build continuing care units, as far as possible, in areas without existing or alternative services. The constraint was usually the preparedness of the local NHS to comply with the Society's conditions. Ipswich was one such area where there was no hospice, but the local health authority in Suffolk would not agree to contribute to such a unit's operating costs. The south-west was another part of the country where the local NHS was unhelpful. The Society, probably wisely, concentrated its efforts on those towns where there was confirmed local NHS support, though it was a matter of much regret that in some areas the local NHS managers were so short-sighted.

On the other hand, despite the standardisation of its approach, the Society was always prepared to consider different solutions if local needs warranted it. One example was Wales. The Society had agreed to support the development of a continuing care unit at the Morriston Hospital in Swansea. Ty Olwen (meaning the House of Olwen) opened in 1981. However, beyond the conurbations of south Wales and the coast of north Wales, the greater part of the principality comprised of isolated rural and mining communities. A full–scale unit in one of these communities would have been quite uneconomic. The Welsh Hospital Board proposed that the Society might support the construction of a number of single–bed, or two–bedded units at several small community hospitals. This would allow for very sick patients to be cared for locally, in familiar surroundings, and without visitors having the arduous travel to a big city.

Henry Garnett met with the hospital board, and agreed the construction of eight two-bed wards extensions to cottage hospitals, six in south Wales and two in the north. These mini–units, as they were called, were not an unqualified success, mainly because of shortfalls in NHS staffing and staff training. However, the principle of providing the service as close as possible to the patient's home was, and remains, a guiding one.

Although the NHS was becoming the Society's chosen partner for hospice development, collaborating with other charities was always another option so long as the Society could avoid any obligation to pay for the long-term operating costs. Capital grants were made to St Joseph's Hospice near Liverpool, to St Ann's Hospice in Manchester for the construction of a second hospice in another part of its catchment area,[9] and to the Community Health Council in Wolverhampton which had been given a lease of Compton Hall for a peppercorn rent for the development of a hospice service.

One of the largest grants, of £100,000, was to the Marie Curie Memorial Foundation to help with the construction of a large home in Glasgow called Hunter's Hill. The Society had long been aware that Glasgow was a cancer black spot, and the new home, with more than forty beds, in the district of Springburn, would make a huge difference to the care of patients. Garnett also set about working with the King Edward VII Hospital in Midhurst. This independent hospital, a former TB sanatorium, was set in a piece of outstandingly beautiful Sussex countryside. Garnett believed, wrongly as it turned out, that a continuing care unit in the hospital would attract sufficient funding from the local NHS to pay its way. The Society paid for the refurbishment of a small ward and, exceptionally, agreed to pay a proportion of the annual operating costs for a fixed period. Unfortunately, financial support from the local NHS never got anywhere near full funding of the service, and it has remained ever since the only hospice inpatient and home care service that the Society funds on a continuing basis.

The other matter that drew Garnett's attention was the Society's policy of making grants towards the operating costs of a handful of voluntary hospices, but only if the hospices made some charge to patients. Garnett at once saw the contradictory position the Society had put itself in. On the one hand the Society was building hospices for the NHS where treatment and care would be given freely irrespective of a patient's income. On the other, the Society was encouraging the voluntary hospices to make charges to patients according to their means. Garnett persuaded the Society to change the basis of their payments towards voluntary hospice running costs. Instead of paying towards the upkeep of poorer patients, the Society agreed, from 1975, to make grants to cover the costs of maintaining a number of inpatient beds – rather like the contractual grants made to voluntary hospices by the NHS. In the case of Copper Cliff, for example, the Society agreed to pay for the cost of maintaining eight of the hospice's beds, or £20,000 per year. This did mean that the Society had to draw a line beneath those hospices already receiving this recurring financial support, and no support of this kind was subsequently agreed for any other voluntary hospice.

Garnett's much-expanded building programme was funded by a series of local appeals, together with the new national appeal recommended by the treasurer and the vice chairman. This dual approach would be repeated again in later years, and the appeal would become one of the Society's standard means of income generation. Local appeals were launched in Southampton to raise funds for the building of Countess Mountbatten House, in Tayside and in Grampian to support the two units named Roxburghe House, in Oxford to help fund Sir Michael Sobell House, and in almost every town where a new continuing care unit was to be built. The Society hoped to raise as much as 50 per cent of the costs of a new building from local people – a figure that was often surpassed.

Running a local appeal was a big job requiring good public relations skills as well as a knowledge of fund-raising. Senior or well-known people from the local community had to be recruited to join an appeal committee, the local newspapers had to be brought on side, and every community group and association encouraged to support the appeal. Since cancer was affecting more and more people, directly or indirectly, an appeal for funds to build a new centre to help very sick cancer patients was an attractive cause for many would-be donors. The programme of local appeals greatly enhanced the local profile and reputation of the Society.

The new national appeal was needed to add to the sum of money that had been raised by the Lillian Board Appeal, most of which was used to fund the unit in Southampton. However, rather than launch another very public national appeal that would compete with the local appeals that were under way, it was decided to mount a low-key campaign that would target grant-giving trusts, industry, commerce and professional associations. The appeal was timed to coincide with the Queen's silver jubilee in 1977.

Henry Garnett and Jocelyn Hambro were able to recruit John King,[10] chairman of the engineering company Babcock & Wilcox, to be chairman of the appeal, and with King came office space in Pall Mall. An experienced appeals director, Noel MacDonald, was appointed to work with King, and provincial committees were set up around the country, but with advice not to cut across the Society's other fund-raising activities. Nearly 500 people attended a fund-raising reception at the Dorchester Hotel hosted by Sir Edwin McAlpine and with future prime minister Margaret Thatcher as the special guest. Meanwhile, the BBC allocated the Society another radio appeal, which was made by the popular actor of the day, Kenneth More. It took about eighteen months for the appeal to reach its target of £1 million, and it finally exceeded the target by more than 10 per cent.

The success of the Society's fund-raising during the 1970s was all the more remarkable when viewed against the backdrop of the nation's economic plight. International financial instability and other adverse economic factors caused in Britain record levels of inflation, sky-high interest rates, industrial dislocation and growing unemployment. In their annual reports for these years, treasurers Jocelyn Hambro and Lord Irwin commented on the inevitable and unavoidable rise in the Society's costs, but they could boast when tight management kept the rises below the year's level of inflation.[11] More importantly, the economic position was having a significant impact on the Society's main partner,

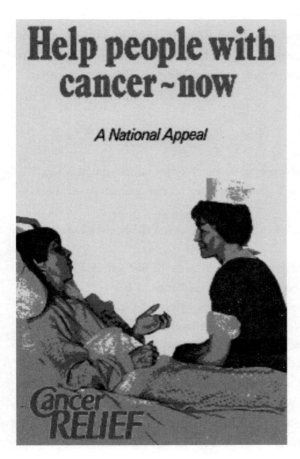

The national appeal.

the National Health Service. The level of public expenditure was a key tool in the government's management of the economy, and the financial crisis meant that it had to be tightly controlled. In the early years of the decade, the amount spent on health services was cash limited but with provision made for inflation. As things worsened, the provision for inflation was abandoned, so the impact of inflation could only be accommodated through efficiency savings or by cutting some part of the service. In these circumstances, regional and area health authorities were very reluctant to agree to any new initiatives that would add to their financial commitments. By early 1980, and with even tougher restrictions in place, Garnett reported that, apart from the units under construction, the Society's buildings programme had come to a halt.

Its partner, the NHS, had simply run out of money. This economic uncertainty would be, as we will see in the next chapter, one of the factors to drive a completely new programme – the Macmillan nurse.

Notes & References

1. Garnett suffered from chest disease for much of his middle and later life.
2. He was 6ft 7in tall, and he began a series, for his two immediate successors were both over 6ft 4in tall.
3. Arrow Enterprises had failed to meet its targets and the Society had terminated its contract.
4. Cicely Saunders died as a patient in the hospice she had founded in 2005.
5. The unit was officially opened by Earl Mountbatten of Burma.
6. She was the grandmother of the late Diana, Princess of Wales.
7. Continuing care is best described as a high level of medical and nursing care required by a patient, but which can be provided outside of the acute hospital setting. In the context of patients with incurable cancer, palliative care is more specific and now more commonly used.
8. Enoch Powell (1912–98) was Minister of Health from 1960 to 1963. Although not remembered for his support for public expenditure, he launched an ambitious ten-year programme of hospital building. *The Hospital Plan for England and Wales* was published in 1962.
9. This was at Little Hulton, near Worsley.
10. He became Sir John King in 1979 and Lord King of Wartnaby in 1983. He was chairman of British Airways from 1981 to 1993. He died in 2005.
11. To give one example, the cost of a standard design continuing care unit rose during the decade from £200,000 to £500,000.

11

The Macmillan Nurse is Born

A workforce of nurses, paid or voluntary, who would care for cancer patients in their own homes was another of Douglas Macmillan's hopes for the future. In fact, a service of this kind had first been provided to patients by the Glasgow Cancer & Skin Institute in the 1890s, but it had not been copied elsewhere. The Society had appointed its own health visitors in the 1930s but they were always few in number and covered only limited areas. The Marie Curie Memorial Foundation launched a home nursing service for patients in London in the early 1950s, but it too was slow to develop and had only twenty-six nurses by 1959. It was not until the growth of modern hospices that cancer nursing at home at last had a wide base for development. At St Christopher's Hospice, Cicely Saunders was among the first to see that good terminal care had to cross the inpatient–outpatient boundary, and in 1969 a service working from the hospice, called home care or domiciliary care, was set up. Other leaders in the rapidly expanding hospice movement were soon to follow.

One of them was Fisher at the Macmillan unit in Christchurch. Henry Garnett attended the official opening of the new unit in 1975 and he came back and reported how impressed he had been to see the domiciliary service based at the unit. Fisher had based the specification for his domiciliary nurses much on the model of the community diabetes nurse. A few months later, the Society gave the unit a further grant of £5,000 per year for two years, in order to add a night nursing service to complement that offered during the day time. The Society's grant was made 'in order to enable [the] unit to provide a complete in-patient and out-patient service to cancer patients within the community, and, in so doing, serve as a yard-stick for Continuing Care Units in the society's … programme'.

Fisher had by now become a member of the Society's governing council and he was keen to encourage the Society to fund more home care projects. He argued that the development of home care nursing 'was of vital importance to the upholding of the standard of care afforded by the [continuing care] units'.

A new service, using Fisher's expertise, was set up alongside the Society's inpatient unit at the King Edward VII Hospital in Midhurst. The Society then received a request from St Joseph's Hospice in Hackney. A young doctor at the hospice, Richard Lamerton, had begun a home care service and was seeking funds to appoint additional nurses to be a part of the team. The Society was keen to support the only hospice in London's East End, where illness and poverty were still way above national averages, and it agreed to make a grant to allow Lamerton to double the number of home care nurses to eight.

At first, Garnett proposed a condition that the nurses funded by the Society should bear the Society's name and be called 'Cancer Relief Nurses'. Garnett, with his businessman's head, together with one or two other leading voices in the Society, was becoming increasingly conscious that the Society received little or no public acknowledgement for the help and support for patients that it was funding. Welfare grants were still being paid anonymously. The continuing care units were named after important supporters or major donors of funds. The Society's payments towards hospice operating costs were not recorded in any way that would attract public attention.

On the other hand, the Society's ability to raise money was obviously linked to how much people knew about the Society's work. By contrast, the Marie Curie Memorial Foundation hospices were called Marie Curie Homes and the nurses, Marie Curie nurses. Homes run by the Sue Ryder Foundation, Dr Barnardo's and the Leonard Cheshire Foundation all bore their charity's name. For the Society, one of its concerns was still that many patients did not know that cancer was their diagnosis, in the widespread belief that unknowing patients would become too distressed if they became aware of the truth.[1]

For this reason, Lamerton had to refuse Garnett's request. The name 'Macmillan' had already been applied collectively to the continuing care units, and it was included in the name of the hospices at Stoke, Christchurch and Midhurst. In internal discussions the Society was already using terms such as 'Macmillan patient care' and 'Macmillan standards'. Garnett therefore proposed to Lamerton that the new home care nurses at St Joseph's Hospice be called Macmillan nurses, and the hospice agreed.[2] The Macmillan nurse, first so called in 1977, would become the most important icon for the Society, and in some ways it would become bigger than the Society itself.

The home care service created by Lamerton, supported by the Society and now bearing the Macmillan name, was soon seen as a standard that should be copied elsewhere. Word about the Society's willingness to fund similar operations quickly got round the hospice world, and the Society was soon asked to support many new schemes. Taking advantage of this opportunity to extend and improve cancer services, all of the early Macmillan services were based at hospices. In 1978 services were established at St Columba's Hospice in Edinburgh, at Sir Michael Sobell House in Oxford and at St Luke's Nursing Home in Sheffield, each of them large hospices in an urban setting.

In Bath, the local charity set up to provide hospice services for cancer patients, the Dorothy House Foundation, faced particular difficulties. It covered a large geographical area, some of which was rural in character. Providing a service to people at home was much more practical, from the point of view of the patients and their families, than in a hospice some miles away and often with inadequate public transport links. The Foundation decided to base its service on domiciliary care, with just a small unit of six inpatient beds for back-up at its centre in Bath. Garnett was impressed with this innovative approach and persuaded the Society to make a substantial investment in the Foundation, about £50,000 per year for three years, so that it could recruit more nurses. Garnett was determined that the scheme 'must not fail for lack of funds'.

Garnett was also impressed with the Foundation's chairman Mrs Prue Clench. Clench was a trained nurse who had developed a keen interest in the care of the dying, and in particular, their care at home. She had written a standard textbook on the subject. After her time at Bath, Garnett recruited her as an adviser to the Society and she played a key role in establishing many of the Society's new Macmillan services.[3] During the year 1981 she held discussions with no less than seventy-three NHS health authorities about the introduction of new Macmillan nurse services.

Ever since Fisher had established the first continuing care unit, or hospice, as an integral part of an NHS service, the Society's preference had been to work with the NHS where possible. In exchange for the Society's funds to build a unit, the NHS would agree to manage and operate the unit and meet all of its year-to-year costs. In setting up the new Macmillan domiciliary services, Garnett also preferred to work with the NHS, and he devised a not dissimilar funding arrangement. The Society agreed to pay for the costs of each domiciliary nurse for a period of three years, in return for the agreement of the NHS to maintain the service subsequently and, critically, to keep the Macmillan name. Even though most of the new domiciliary services were being based at voluntary hospices, Garnett still tried to negotiate and secure their long-term funding with the NHS wherever possible. The logic of this approach was that new Macmillan services did not have to be linked to hospices at all, but rather they could be set up as part of hospital and district nursing services.

NHS managers also saw this opportunity. By the end of 1981 there were thirty-five domiciliary Macmillan nursing services up and running across Great Britain. Eight of these were at Macmillan continuing care units built for the NHS and nineteen were based at voluntary hospices. Macmillan nursing services had also been established at the hospital in Bridgend, at King's College Hospital in south-east London, at the Royal Hallamshire Hospital in Sheffield, and at the district hospital in Eastbourne. In addition, Macmillan domiciliary services complemented the care for patients offered at the mini-units in Wales.

Domiciliary care was becoming as important as inpatient care, if not more so. The fact that most patients preferred to be cared for at home was well known. Unless their home circumstances are particularly unsatisfactory, people with terminal illness will usually be happier to remain at home in familiar surroundings and with close relatives and friends, if that is at all possible. Moreover, according to Professor Eric Wilkes, 'more people are admitted to a hospice because of the needs of their family, than ever their own'.[4]

Wilkes's point was that it was the carers at home who often needed help and support to look after very sick relatives, and that so long as this help and support could be given, so many more patients could remain at home and, indeed, could die at home. Wilkes was appointed chairman of a DHSS working party to consider the future of the care of the dying and he concluded that:

Terminal care is not a matter of new buildings or expensive equipment. … Our objective now should be to ensure that every dying patient has access to professional staff who can provide the appropriate care.

The way forward is to encourage the dissemination of the principles of terminal care throughout the health service …

Wilkes's report was welcomed by government and it had an important impact on the Society. It was the springboard from which the domiciliary Macmillan nurse programme, particularly within the NHS, could develop and expand beyond early expectation. As the Society's 75th anniversary report said:

Despite the practical and emotional demands of caring for a dying patient at home, most families have the strength and the courage to cope, provided they have the right support. Giving this support is the role of the Macmillan nurse …

Wilkes argued for no further hospice building and increasingly it was accepted that the inpatient hospice should be there as a back-up to the domiciliary care service, rather than the other way round. The inpatient hospice should be there for patients who, because of the complications of their illness or their home circumstances, could not be cared for at home. Accordingly, Garnett reported to the Society's council (in September 1980) that: 'It was now generally agreed that continuing care units should be centres of excellence and teaching, and that domiciliary care should, as far as possible, be extended on a nationwide basis.'

This strategic approach to providing palliative care for cancer patients found much favour within the Department of Health and Social Security and the NHS, not only because of the patient centred solution it proposed, but also because it was much less costly than operating more inpatient hospices. The tight rein on public expenditure imposed during the second half of the 1970s had been pulled back even further with the election of the Conservative government of Margaret Thatcher in 1979. Her first Secretary of State for Health and Social Security, Patrick Jenkin, declared in the government's policy document, *Care in Action*,[5] that 'the Government's top priority must be to get the economy right; for that reason, it cannot be assumed that more money will always be available to be spent on health care'.

Wilkes had understood that sufficient funds would just not be available, from any sources, to pay for every patient to be cared for in a hospice, and in any event, he questioned their cost effectiveness. To a Society-sponsored seminar[6] he said:

We, in [St Luke's Nursing Home] Sheffield, look after something like ten per cent of all local cancer deaths; but that does not really excuse an outlay of £300,000 a year to look after 400 dying patients a year ... there is no hope of providing such support for all.

Wilkes went on to stress that,

no area health authority can nowadays gladly accept the revenue consequences of a specialist [hospice] unit no matter how highly desirable.

The era of inpatient hospice construction was over, at least within the NHS. Government policy, as outlined in *Care in Action*, was to encourage care in the community as a more patient orientated and less costly alternative to care as an inpatient.

The strategies of the government and of the Society thereby became congruent, with the result that there was a huge growth in the number of Macmillan domiciliary nursing services over the following years. Garnett said: 'This venture into domiciliary care will re-awaken interest in those who have been frustrated by present financial restrictions in their desire to build a hospice.'

By the end of 1983 there were 205 Macmillan nurses in post, and two years later there were more than 330, working in 120 teams throughout Britain. The 500th Macmillan nurse[7] was appointed in 1988 to work at Newcastle General Hospital. According to Stephanie Morgan, a Macmillan nurse working from the King Edward VII Hospital in Midhurst,[8] the patient care of a Macmillan domiciliary service had four main objectives:

> to improve the quality of [a patient's] remaining life by the elimination of pain or the control of symptoms,
> to help maintain [a patient's] independence and dignity,
> to give [a patient] opportunities to talk about feelings aroused by the disease and the prognosis, [and]
> to help the patient remain in his (or her) own home, with its continuing family relationships, until the end, if this is desired and possible.

All domiciliary Macmillan nurses, apart from being state-registered nurses[9], had to hold a district nurse or health visitor's qualification, and they had to have undertaken a specialist course in the nursing care of the dying. As specialists in the care of terminally ill patients (the vast majority of whom would be dying from cancer), Macmillan nurses were able to offer a patient, and his or her family, expert help, information and advice about all aspects of their care, emotional support, and links into social services. Most importantly, the Macmillan nurse had the time to talk to a patient and his or her family, and to listen to the patient's feelings and fears. The spread of Macmillan services throughout the UK brought about a radical improvement in the care that terminally ill cancer patients at home could expect.

The early Macmillan nurses had no ready-prepared protocols by which to work. They were breaking new ground. One of the first nurses to be appointed, Ann Nash, recalled, 'The future was uncertain, but the opportunity was too exciting to miss. We learned on our feet.'[10]

Often, the nurses' first task would be to find themselves some office space, a filing cabinet, a telephone, and some secretarial help. In the early times, they could be on call for 24 hours a day, and for seven days a week. It was work that could be exhausting both physically and emotionally, but also very rewarding. As one nurse said:

> ... as a Macmillan nurse you know that you are giving the best you can. You have more time to give to your patient and to the family. You have more time to spare [for them], and more knowledge to share.

And another said:

> I love my work. There is something so satisfying about helping people through a very bad time and knowing that those who are left will be sad but never broken.

The early Macmillan nurses, whether based at hospices or in hospitals and clinics, had to build good relationships with general practitioners, district nurses and other health care professionals who could be defensive, and even antagonistic, to the suggestion that more could be done for their terminally ill patients. The problem was well put by Dr Derek Doyle, the medical director of St Columba's Hospice in Edinburgh. He said in 1980[11] that,

> Until a relatively few years ago one had to be guarded and diplomatic when explaining to an audience of doctors ... why a special ... care programme was needed for the dying. ... That many of us had inadequate training on the subject was usually accepted, but quickly countered with the comment that our post-graduate experience had more than made up for this deficiency.

These were the words of a senior and much respected doctor. A newly appointed nurse trying to convince a sceptical doctor would have a doubly difficult task. Nevertheless, by patience and perseverance, and by a daily demonstration of their value, the Macmillan nurses became more and more accepted. Prue Clench and another Macmillan nursing advisor, Barbara Dicks, soon played an important part preparing standard operational policies and briefing materials for NHS health authorities and other professional staff.

The expansion of domiciliary Macmillan nursing was also helped by Rita O'Brien, who Garnett had cleverly recruited from the Department of Health and Social Security with a brief to develop new Macmillan services. O'Brien had been the principal in the department responsible for cancer and terminal care policy, and so had a very wide range of contacts within the NHS. She was strongly committed to improving the care of patients in the public sector. In 1985 she could report proudly that:

> Macmillan Home Care Nurses were now widely regarded ... as the most significant contribution yet made by [the Society] to improving the care of cancer patients. The Macmillan nurse took the skills developed in the hospices and continuing care units out into the community. ... This meant that far more people had access to specialist care.

O'Brien went on to estimate that it would be possible to have Macmillan nurses covering much of the country within five years.

Wilkes's challenge to spread good palliative care throughout the NHS was comprehensive and it embraced more than hospice and home. Most patients dying of cancer were (and still are) cared for in hospital, and often on general medical and surgical wards. Few medical or nursing staff would have any specialist knowledge or skills in caring for the dying. Garnett would quote figures that 60 per cent of all deaths each year occurred in hospitals, and that only 18 per cent of them with terminal illness got proper care. One big step forward was the recruitment of Macmillan nurses to work with patients being cared for on hospital wards and those attending hospital as outpatients. The concept of a 'hospital support team' for the terminally ill had been pioneered at St Thomas's Hospital in London by Dr Thelma Bates, who had learned her skills at St Christopher's Hospice. By the end of the 1980s, Macmillan nurse services had been set up in more than twenty hospitals, including many in cities with high rates of cancer deaths such as Liverpool, Derby, Hull and Leeds.

As the number of Macmillan nurses increased, so did the need to train them. Fisher began to invite newly appointed nurses to undertake training at his unit in Christchurch as early as 1976. Soon, courses were also offered at the units in Oxford and Southampton. The standard course for a nurse specialising in the care of the terminally ill was run under the direction of the English National Board for Nursing and Midwifery Studies.[12] It was a six-week course, usually taught at a hospice, and covered both the care of the dying patient and the patient's family. A more advanced course later became available.

The number of courses offered, and the number of places available on each course was very limited, and nurses would often have to wait many months, sometimes even more than a year, to get a place. The Society responded by encouraging and funding the development of teaching centres at the Macmillan continuing care units and at voluntary hospices. Garnett regarded each Macmillan unit as a potential centre of excellence and he encouraged them to link up with nearby universities. On top of the basic and advanced courses, the Society began also to hold regular seminars for Macmillan nurses, partly to keep them up to date, but also to give them the opportunity to meet with each other.

The rapid growth of Macmillan nursing services needed an equally rapid growth of income to pay for them and for their training. John King's appeal had been for the Macmillan continuing care units, and the regular income from local committees and other fund-raising activities would not be sufficient to fund an ambitious programme of new nurses. Another appeal was needed, and the task of planning and organising it fell to the Society's appeals committee, chaired by Hugh Dundas.[13] Dundas had first become involved with the Society in 1976. He was chairman of the services company BET and of Thames Television, and he had a wide circle of business contacts. He was also a much decorated fighter pilot from the Second World War, and a man of enormous charm and ability.

In 1982 the second national appeal was launched, with a target of £3 million. Dundas's plan was to recruit a number of influential people from all over the country and to get them to make approaches to potential donors. A press launch came in the September at which a film

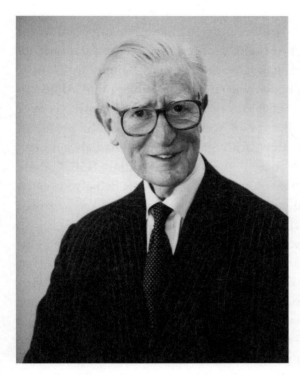

Sir Hugh Dundas.

about the Society's work, *Help People Now*, was shown. It was probably not a coincidence that the launch was well covered by, among other media, Thames Television. This appeal was not a complete success, and it was closed after it had raised about £2 million. Dundas had realised that people preferred to give to local appeals where the funds would be used to improve local cancer care services, and he recommended that a programme of local appeals become a regular part of fund-raising activity. This advice was heeded and local appeals were, for many years, the most prominent aspect of the Society's local fund-raising, often greatly exceeding their targets. In 1986 an appeals manager, Simon Lloyd, was appointed to give them direction and coordination. Lloyd, an old colleague of Garnett's from the Gillette company, set about reorganising and strengthening the Society's regional structures so that they could cope with what Lloyd called this 'explosion' of activity. And the explosion was not restricted to Macmillan nurses. There were other things that had to be paid for.

The success of the Macmillan nurse had another implication for the Society, or at least it brought another issue to the fore. Despite all that it was doing in cancer care, the National Society for Cancer Relief remained a little-known charity in the public mind. Although one of the oldest cancer charities in the country, all those years of near anonymity meant that it had nothing like the public profile of the cancer research charities. Although the Society had always been known in shorthand as Cancer Relief, or by its initials NSCR, these were really for internal use only. Grants to patients had always been paid anonymously, and the words *cancer relief* were not linked to any of the Society's newer activities.

Instead, the title 'Macmillan' was now being used as a prefix to describe the Society's patient services. With the enormous success of the Macmillan nurse, far more people recognised the words 'Macmillan nurse' than they ever did 'National Society for Cancer Relief', or 'Cancer Relief'. This inevitably inhibited fund-raising, since there was no charity called the 'Macmillan nurses' for people to donate to. The Society decided to change its name for a second time. From 1983 the Society became known publicly as the Macmillan Cancer Relief Fund, and then the following year as the Cancer Relief Macmillan Fund. The shorthand name of Cancer Relief survived for a few years more and the initials CRMF also came into use. However, increasingly, the shorthand name 'Macmillan' began to be used.[14] For the remainder of this book, the Society will be called Macmillan, the shorthand name by which it is known today.

Notes & References

1. One patient, known to the author, who had undergone laryngectomy for a malignant growth in 1988 was told by his doctor that he had a tumour in the throat, whereupon the patient said to his family with relief that 'at least it is not cancer!'
2. This account is confirmed both by Richard Lamerton in *A Bit of Heaven for the Few, An oral history of the hospice movement in the United Kingdon*, published by Observatory Publications in 2005, and by Joan Bebbington, who worked

closely with Garnett at the time, in conversation with the author on 6 June 2005.

3. Clench was author of *Managing to Care, community services for the terminally ill*, published by Patten Press in 1984. She died of cancer in 2004 aged 62.

4. Wilkes was Professor of Community Care and General Practice at the University of Sheffield 1971–84 and the first medical director of St Luke's Nursing Home in Sheffield. He made this point on many occasions.

5. Published by the DHSS in 1981.

6. Report of the Macmillan Seminar on Domiciliary Care, held on 5–7 December 1980 at Milton Hill House, Abingdon, published in 1981 by NSCR.

7. Maureen Laverty.

8. Article in *The Medical Practitioner.*

9. The qualification of State Registered Nurse (SRN) was the standard qualification for nurses before the introduction of the Registered General Nurse (RGN) qualification.

10. Cancer Relief Macmillan Fund Review, 1988–9.

11. Macmillan Seminar, 5–7 December 1980.

12. The board was wound up in 2002 and its responsibilities transferred to the new Nursing & Midwifery Council.

13. Later, Sir Hugh Dundas. He died of cancer in 1995.

14. This found little favour with the other Macmillan, the very well-known publishing house founded in 1843 by Harold Macmillan's grandfather. Many years later, a friendly accommodation was reached between the publisher and the charity about the shared use of the name.

12

Education and Consolidation

The rapid growth of Macmillan services for inpatients and outpatients was just one part of the major expansion of medical and nursing services for the incurably or terminally ill pioneered by Cicely Saunders, and which spread across the United Kingdom, albeit haphazardly, and then to the Anglo-Saxon world and beyond. By the early seventies it was being called palliative care, because its purpose was to palliate or relieve, but not cure.[1] A comprehensive, but succinct, description of the discipline comes from Twycross and Miller:

> Palliative care is far more than symptom relief. It addresses physical, psychological, social and spiritual aspects of suffering, thereby helping patients to come to terms with their impending death as constructively as they can while living as actively and creatively as possible. Palliative care also provides a parallel support system to help families cope during the patient's illness and a bereavement; it is best provided by a multi-professional team.[2]

Within that second sentence is a very big bundle of professional skills, and hence the condition in the last, that good palliative care needs many different hands.

Medical care is, of course, absolutely fundamental to good palliative care. A patient who is suffering with pain or other distressing symptoms cannot possibly cope well with his or her remaining weeks or months of life, but this was the picture that Saunders and her fellow practitioners saw only too often on the wards of NHS (and private) hospitals. There was not infrequently reluctance on the part of doctors to administer the most powerful painkilling drugs – the opioids[3] – or to give them in sufficient doses to be continuously effective. Moreover, other symptoms, such as nausea, vomiting, constipation, breathing difficulties and problems with swallowing – inevitable and unavoidable consequences of the disease process and often bringing as much wretchedness as pain – were similarly not effectively treated.

The doctors who now specialised in palliative medicine, still mostly working in hospices, had developed drug regimes and advanced techniques of treatments that could maintain most patients free from pain and relatively free from other debilitating symptoms through the whole terminal period. With this expert medical care came the need for equally skilled nursing. The nurse who specialised in the care of the dying would have a substantial knowledge of the progress of the disease, the possible or likely symptoms to come, the treatment options and their side effects, and the particular implications and complications of different cancers. Indeed, Douglas Scott, Garnett's later successor, recalled that the average Macmillan nurse would see 100 new cases of cancer every year, while the average general practitioner would see just five.

With this experience on top of basic nursing skills, the specialist nurse could give the patient, and the patient's family, expert help and support, enabling them to cope with the disease and allay unwarranted fears. For some patients, the help of a physiotherapist might be needed in addition, to overcome physical disability caused by the progress or treatment of the cancer. For others, where there were particular family problems, the input of the local social services team was called for. The emotional or psychological care of patients and their families was also important. Depression or overwhelming anguish is not uncommon in the dying.

All professional carers need to have some knowledge of counselling to help patients express their fears, and for some patients or close relatives more radical intervention, even from a psychiatrist, might be needed. For bereaved relatives, this support might be required for months or even years after the patient's death. The role of the spiritual minister was also still important to many, be they Christians, Muslims, Jews or members of other communities of faith.

Spreading this knowledge about palliative care and the skills that were required throughout the National Health Service, as Wilkes had called for, was an enormous task and it is doubtful if it has been achieved even as this book is written thirty or more years on. It could only be accomplished if two things were in place. First, there had to be sufficient training opportunities available so that doctors, nurses and the other professionals working with the terminally ill, wherever they may be, could receive the necessary tuition. Given that patients with terminal cancer can be cared for in almost any hospital or nursing home, and within every GP practice, this amounted to a very large number of people who needed to be offered some education or training. Second, the powerful professional groups in the NHS, the doctors and the nurses, had to be a part of the plan. The quotation from Doyle in the last chapter gave some indication that the task would be a big one. Moreover, the most urgent need was to provide sufficiently well-qualified staff, and particularly doctors, to fill all the posts in the Macmillan units and hospices, and to support the hospital teams. The programme of nurse training had already begun in the 1970s and, in 1980, Macmillan began its support for medical training. It started by offering bursaries to doctors wishing to improve their skills through training at a Macmillan continuing care unit. This was followed by a programme of funding medical education programmes set up by hospices.

Macmillan was able to recruit to its council several senior medical and nurse practitioners who would use their influence and offer advice in developing programmes of training. Wilkes himself was a member of the council until 1984, and other well-known names included the doctors Fisher, Doyle and Hillier.

At the beginning, Macmillan's education programme was slow to start and it lacked focus and drive. In late 1982 the Reverend

Tom Scott, the founder and manager of Strathcarron Hospice near Falkirk, joined Macmillan on a part-time basis as executive officer for Scotland. Scott was a man of great vision who had decided to take his Christian ministry to the care of the dying, and he would play an important role in the society, both in Scotland and across the UK, for the next fifteen years.[4]

Scott believed passionately in spreading the best palliative and terminal care throughout the NHS, and he soon became chairman of the Macmillan patient care committee and the leading advocate of an education strategy. But Scott was wise, and he understood that Macmillan had to work closely with professional groups and the NHS if it was to be effective. The result was the setting up of the Macmillan Education Unit in the Department of Pharmacology and Therapeutics at the Royal London Hospital Medical School. The unit worked with the counsel and advice of an education and training panel and a nursing panel, both of which included many people from outside Macmillan. The head of the unit was Jennifer Raiman, a senior educationalist and researcher, who easily crossed the professional boundaries between doctors and nurses and other professional groups. Raiman had been responsible for the London Hospital Pain Observation Chart which became a standard tool for use in the NHS. She later became Macmillan's Head of Medical Services, and remained with Macmillan until 1996. Scott and Raiman worked together to develop the Macmillan education programme.

Raiman's unit at the Royal London Hospital was supported by Dr Ray Corcoran, the senior medical tutor at St Joseph's Hospice; by Edward Monypenny, a surgeon from St Giles' Hospice in Lichfield; and by Prue Clench. Professor Duncan Vere of the hospital's medical school acted as chairman. Other experts joined the unit later. It began to produce a range of professional and academic materials and data to support those teaching terminal care. According to Raiman, the unit was concerned with answering the key questions of 'how to teach, what to teach, whom to teach, [and] how to know the teaching is effective'.

Importantly, the unit's advice and support were available to all the voluntary hospices providing teaching, as well as the continuing care homes funded by Macmillan and operating within the NHS. This initiative was followed in Scotland by a partnership with the Centre for

Medical Education at the University of Dundee to produce distance learning materials in terminal care for doctors and other professionals, and later for general practitioners. To be really effective, however, the major thrust of the education programme had to be with the funding of teaching posts.

Jennifer Raiman and Tom Scott announced Macmillan's long-term education strategy in 1985. Its central plank was to support a series of Macmillan lecturer-ships at medical and nursing schools across the UK. According to Scott, this plan was to help not only doctors and nurses working in the Macmillan homes, but for all those who in their day-to-day practice had to care for people with terminal cancer. The first post agreed was at Dundee, where the lecturer, Dr Martin Leiper, would concentrate on teaching the control of pain and other symptoms of terminal illness on courses lasting between three and six months. The second post was for a lecturer in the nursing care of the terminally ill based at King's College Hospital in London. The appointee was Jessica Corner, who later held professorships at London and Southampton universities, and who then became a trustee of Macmillan; later still she became the charity's Director of Improving Cancer Services.

Posts followed at the universities of Southampton, Birmingham, Oxford, Leeds, Manchester and Glasgow. In all, eleven academic posts were planned, though some post-holders were diverted into clinical work at the expense of teaching. In addition, fourteen new nurse tutor posts were programmed and early appointments were made at Sheffield, Wolverhampton and Bath. Most of the posts were approved with guaranteed funding from Macmillan for five years. In 1980 Macmillan spent nearly £25,000 on education. By 1986 this figure had grown nearly six-fold to £465,000,[5] and by the end of the decade it had risen to nearly £1 million.

Apart from the obvious impact the academic teaching programme had in terms of raising standards of patient care, it had another, and very important, result. It played a part in elevating the status of palliative care in the professional and academic worlds. The Royal College of Nursing set up its own specialist forum on palliative care, and in 1987 the Royal College of Physicians recognised palliative medicine as a medical speciality in its own right, ranking it with geriatrics, paediatrics, oncology etc. This made the discipline a more attractive career option for young doctors. Doyle and others had been arguing for some time that palliative medicine should have this status, but the College could not have agreed without the accredited university graduate and postgraduate courses in the subject that had become available, so many of them financed by Macmillan.

A secondary line of work, but another of strategic necessity, was to address the shortage of fully skilled medical practitioners to fill the new permanent posts in palliative medicine that were becoming available. Macmillan started a series of initiatives to tackle the problem. Macmillan fellowships were introduced to enable young doctors working in hospitals or in community services to extend their training into palliative medicine, and even to take some formal qualification in the discipline. Macmillan registrar posts were established to give more senior doctors the opportunity to practise palliative medicine, probably for the first time, under the direction of a consultant. The first posts were allocated to Countess Mountbatten House in Southampton and to St Columba's Hospice in Edinburgh, and others followed in Aberdeen, Birmingham, London, Nottingham and elsewhere. Palliative medicine within NHS hospitals was further boosted by the appointment of Macmillan consultants who, working with their colleagues in other disciplines, could give advice and support for the care of the terminally ill.

The medical education programme was ambitious, but it could only have a really comprehensive approach if it also tackled the training needs of general practitioners.

Dr David Percy was a Hampshire general practitioner and a clinical assistant at Countess Mountbatten House in Southampton. Here is his discourse on the typical GP's experience of cancer.[6]

In the course of a year, I see about 500 patients with upper respiratory infections, 250 with skin diseases, 200 with emotional disorders and 50 with acute back disorders. I see seven patients with myocardial infarction, five with stroke and five with appendicitis.

What about cancers? First the *rare* tumours. In a year I will see one, perhaps 2 patients with cancer of the lung; one with breast cancer; two bowel cancers every 3 years; and one stomach cancer every two years.

The second group are the *very rare* tumours. Only once in 7 years can I expect to see a patient with cancer of the oesophagus, and every 5 years a patient with ovarian cancer.

The third group are the *extremely rare* tumours – a brain tumour in every ten years or a thyroid cancer in 20 years.

Percy illustrated so well how difficult it was, and doubtless still is, for general practitioners to maintain their skills and knowledge to cover all the cancers that they just might see in a lifetime of practice. The palliative treatment needed for a particular cancer is of course unique to that cancer, and it is also unique to the particular patient.

Few GPs were able to attend lengthy courses on palliative medicine held at one of the Macmillan units or at a hospice (although many one or two day seminars were successfully held). One answer was to take the teaching to the GPs. Macmillan lecturer Martin Leiper at Dundee began to work on a distance learning programme that would enable busy doctors to learn at a time and a place that suited them. The education programme was called MACPAC, abbreviated from Macmillan Palliation in Advanced Cancer. It was a visual and audio computer programme with a supporting manual, and was first launched in 1989. Many GPs were able to make good use of the MACPAC programme, and its success prompted Macmillan to develop MACPAC programmes for hospital doctors and for palliative care nurses.

To complement the Macmillan-funded education and training offered in academic and clinical settings, Macmillan also developed its own programme of seminars for doctors, nurses and other professional groups. These were usually held over a weekend at a residential conference centre. There were seminars for newly appointed Macmillan nurses, experienced Macmillan nurses, Macmillan nurse managers, Macmillan-funded doctors, Macmillan lecturers and social workers. The purpose of the programme was to add to the skills and knowledge of the Macmillan post-holders attending, but also to give them the opportunity to meet with their peers and to discuss matters of mutual interest and concern. In 1990 a total of eighteen weekend seminars were held, nine of them for nurses, and attended by 1,250 practitioners, of whom 670 were nurses.

The success of the strategies initiated by Henry Garnett, including the developments of Macmillan continuing care buildings, the Macmillan nurse, and Macmillan education programmes, reached their zenith in later years. Meanwhile, they increased year by year the size and influence of the charity. Charitable hospices getting off the ground sought financial support from Macmillan for commissioning grants, new domiciliary nursing services and education and training projects, and Macmillan developed an ever closer relationship with the National Health Service. According to Garnett: 'This valuable relationship [had] given the NHS the opportunity to assume its proper role in the care of the terminally ill both in the home and on hospital sites.'

In other words, Macmillan's work was helping the NHS to expand and improve its range of services for those dying of cancer and to live up to the expectation that it would provide medical and health care from the cradle to the grave. In 1985 a conference was convened in London by the Department of Health and Social Security and the National Association of Health Authorities to discuss the future of terminal care provision. The Prince of Wales opened the conference and other speakers included Dame Cicely Saunders and Professor Wilkes. The Minister of State for Health, Barney Hayhoe MP, spoke of the need for health authorities to realise their obligations to dying patients and to draw up comprehensive plans to meet their needs. This was precisely what Macmillan wanted to hear, with Garnett able to respond that: 'We continue to work with Health Authorities, setting up new nursing services [and] helping them plan and finance their day and in-patient units. ... Our aim is to help the NHS to do this wherever we can.'

Macmillan's influence was not universally liked by other charities in the sector, and Garnett recognised that Macmillan's closeness to the NHS was not always conducive to the charity working more closely with the voluntary hospices. Controversially, many voluntary hospices received little or no funding from their local NHS health authorities even though they were caring, free of charge, for NHS patients. There was also frequent conflict between voluntary hospices and local health authorities over their respective plans for the expansion of palliative care services. Some tension was beginning to build between Macmillan and the voluntary hospices which would later lead, in some quarters, even to hostility.

At the same time, Garnett was far from happy when others tried to increase their influence. Garnett was totally committed to Macmillan and to its strategic objectives. In 1984 the Duchess of Norfolk and the British Medical Association founded a charity called Help the Hospices with a brief to raise funds for voluntary hospices and generally to improve the standard and availability of terminal care. Garnett and many of his colleagues were apprehensive about the new initiative. Garnett feared that Help the Hospices would encourage new voluntary hospice building and therefore cut across Macmillan's strategy of strengthening services within the NHS and giving greater emphasis to domiciliary care services. Even the new charity's name, with an implication that it was to support buildings, was worrying. Garnett was alarmed that more resources might be channelled into financing inpatient care, especially if that might be at the cost of home care and the expansion of Macmillan services. Garnett tried to persuade the duchess to abandon the idea, and instead to support Macmillan's fund-raising work. He also used the influence he had with key players in the hospice movement to speak against the new venture but his success was short term. As it turned out, Wilkes became a trustee of the new charity and an influential voice, and he helped to guide it towards an inclusive approach to terminal care covering hospice, hospital and home. Help the Hospices survived and would indeed flourish,[7] although its relationship with Macmillan was strained for a little time. This was a further sign that Macmillan and the growing hospice movement would not always see eye to eye.

Garnett's passion and commitment always lay with Macmillan and with the Macmillan services it had created. He was intensely loyal. At the time of the 1985 conference, Garnett was 72 years of age. He was as energetic as ever but, with his continuing chest illness, retirement had to loom ahead. It was time for him to bow out. At the end of 1986 he decided to stand down as chief executive as soon as a successor had been appointed. This was a felicitous time because it coincided with Macmillan's 75th anniversary, which ran for twelve months from 1 July 1986. The celebration was used to make the public more aware of Macmillan and its work, and of course to raise more funds. But it also allowed for some reflection on what had been achieved, and it would have been impossible to argue with Garnett when he said that, 'Douglas

Macmillan would have been proud to see the way in which his vision of a whole new approach to the care and treatment of cancer patients has been recognised and put into practice'.

Garnett had been the dominant figure in the society for nearly fifteen years, and it is fair to say that more had been achieved in his time than in Macmillan's previous sixty years. Douglas Macmillan would indeed have been proud. Garnett died in October 1990. Ronald Fisher, who had worked with Garnett so closely, wrote of him in the society's newsletter:

> He was most selfless in his devotion to his work. ... I admired his negotiating skills, patience and tact as he gave advice and encouragement. As a result he became well-liked and respected at all levels ... [he] was able to fulfil those dreams [of Douglas Macmillan] and add new dimensions to the name Macmillan.

His obituary in *The Times*[8] said that the Macmillan nurse, 'perhaps above all else, deserves to be his memorial'.

Appropriately, some years later, Macmillan introduced an award for Macmillan nurses who had served with distinction, and called it the Henry Garnett Medal.

Macmillan's new chief executive[9] took up his post in the spring of 1987. He was Douglas Scott, a scion of the Scottish aristocracy[10] with as great a passion for improving the care of people with cancer as Garnett's. Like Garnett, Scott had been schooled at Eton and Sandhurst, and he had spent his early years in the Irish Guards, leaving with the rank of captain. Then, also like Garnett, Scott went into business, working as an executive with the engineering company the TI Group, and later with PE Consulting. Unlike Garnett, Douglas Scott knew all about the ravages of cancer from personal and painful experience. His only son Adam had died of the disease just before his 8th birthday, and Scott himself had had a malignant tumour in his leg removed by surgery in 1984.

Never without a walking stick, cancer left Scott with a profound limp. Highly intelligent, often mercurial, never without audacity and sometimes with a good pinch of hauteur, Scott was steadfast in his allegiance to Macmillan and to the development of more Macmillan services.[11] He was an inspirational leader and hugely popular with his

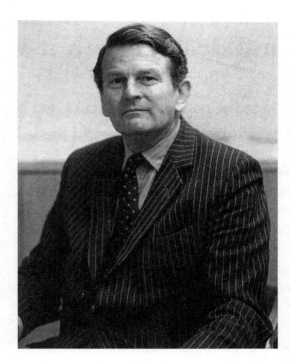

Douglas Scott.

colleagues. Scott was determined to drive Macmillan forward, and he did so until he reached his retirement age in 1995.

Garnett had left for Scott a strong and vibrant organisation on which to build, and a group of very committed people to support him. In 1984 the Countess of Westmorland had been elected as the new president. She was an inspired choice. She had begun her work for charity back in 1955 when she became a voluntary worker in London's East End and first president of the Stars' Organisation for Spastics. In 1981 she became a social worker at the Charing Cross Hospital, and it was through this work that she first became aware of the particular problems and needs of people with cancer. The countess was a hardworking and most charming figurehead for Macmillan until she stood down in 1990.

In 1983 Richard Hambro had been elected treasurer in succession to the Earl of Halifax. Richard, the second son of Jocelyn Hambro, also had very personal reasons which brought him into Macmillan. He had seen his mother Sylvia die of lung cancer just days before Christmas in 1972, and this only nine months after her brother had died of the disease.

Then eleven years later, as we know, his stepmother Elisabeth also died from the disease. Garnett himself had been elected chairman after the death of Elisabeth Hambro, and he continued to hold this position until 1988. He was succeeded by Sir Hugh Dundas.

Macmillan's paid staff also included many of high ability and commitment. As well as Rita O'Brien, Simon Lloyd, Jennifer Raiman and Tom Scott, Garnett had recruited some other very capable people. One was Susan Butler who was responsible for press and public relations. In her thirties with two young children, her feminine demeanour belied a tough and assertive approach. A professional to her fingertips, she was the catalyst behind Macmillan's very successful press and advertising campaigns. Another was Derek Spooner. Recruited from the National Health Service to take control of the building programme, Spooner soon renewed Macmillan's approach to construction and introduced quality as a hallmark of the Macmillan continuing care units.[12] In Scotland, Catherine Duthie, a serious-minded and very effective organiser, had been appointed to manage the society's office. Douglas Scott would later add to the team as Macmillan developed further and its scope grew wider and deeper. One of his first appointments was that of Jeanette Webber to the newly created post of Chief Nursing Adviser. Webber was a very experienced practitioner and educator who carried much influence beyond Macmillan.

There was one final piece of consolidation. Despite the adaptations to the building at Dorset Square, the head office was just too small to accommodate any longer the size of organisation that Macmillan had become. A search was made for new premises, and in due course suitable offices were found in a small block in Britten Street, just off the King's Road in Chelsea. With the agreement of Macmillan's great benefactor Sir Michael Sobell, the Dorset Square building was sold, and the move to Chelsea took place early in 1986. Anchor House was to be the home of Macmillan for the next fourteen years.

Notes & References

1. In fact, the term 'palliative care' was first used in Quebec in Canada, because the words 'hospice care', used by Saunders, would be confused by French speakers with the medieval hospices in France.

2. Chapter on *Palliative Care* by Robert Twycross and Mary Miller, Oxford Textbook of Medicine, 4th edn, 2003.

3. Drugs derived from opium; including morphine, diamorphine (heroin), methadone and pethidine.

4. Tom Scott also maintained close links with hospices through the Association of Hospice Administrators.

5. In the same period, education as a percentage of all money spent on Macmillan's charitable work increased from 1.5 per cent to 7.75 per cent.

6. Macmillan Seminar on Domiciliary Care, held on 5–7 December 1980 at Milton Hill House, Abingdon.

7. In fact, new charitable hospices continued to be built during the 1980s and into the 1990s as groups of volunteers became determined to see the services of St Christopher's Hospice available in their locality. Help the Hospices played no significant part in encouraging them.

8. 22 October 1990.

9. At first his designation was director and general secretary.

10. Scott's father was a grandson of the 6th Duke of Buccleuch, and his mother was the second daughter of Field Marshal Earl Haig, the British commander of the First World War. His full name is Douglas Andrew Montagu Douglas Scott.

11. The writer recalls Scott being interviewed by a journalist working for a charity journal. The journalist asked Scott what had brought about his commitment to the voluntary sector. Scott was scathing in his reply. He said he had no commitment at all to the voluntary sector, but that his only commitment was to Macmillan.

12. Spooner was awarded the OBE for his work in 2001.

13

Bright Patches in the Sky

For the first half a century or more of its existence, Macmillan had worked against a cancer backdrop that was all too pessimistic. Indeed, as the years went on, the picture appeared to become bleaker rather than more positive. Up until Douglas Macmillan's retirement, the annual reports for most years would faithfully record the past year's cancer deaths statistics and, just as faithfully, they would show another rise. For England and Wales, the figures rose from nearly 50,000 deaths per annum in the early 1920s to nearly 90,000 per annum thirty years later. Putting it another way, during this period, the number of people dying from cancer rose from one in 12 of all deaths, to one in 6.[1] As a statistician, Douglas Macmillan was at pains to explain the difference between actual death rates and adjusted rates, taking into account age distribution and other factors, but whichever figures were used the trend was distinctly upwards. As well as being a statistic of great significance for those responsible for the nation's health care, cancer mortality had become a direct and tragic experience for almost every family in the country. The phrase 'everyone knows someone who has, or who has had cancer' had a great deal of resonance.

The promises of surgery and radium treatment, about which there had been much excitement, were slow to realise. It is true that improved operating techniques, better control of patient shock, and blood transfusion had made long and deep surgical operations possible. From the 1930s onward, even the removal of a whole lung became a procedure with a 50-50 chance of recovery. But for the most part, surgery could only be curative if the cancer was discovered in its very early stages, and this happened too rarely in so many types of cancer.

The disease, in these earliest stages tends not to be accompanied by striking symptoms, or indeed, by any symptoms at all. In 1943 mass-radiography was introduced for the early detection of tuberculosis and it would also uncover malignant tumours of the throat, lung and oesophagus. However, only a very small number of cases so found were operable. On top of this, researchers had a much better understanding of how cancers spread from a primary site to other organs. They had originally thought that cancer spread slowly outwards from the first growth and that the body's lymphatic system was the channel of travel to other parts of the body. Cancerous cells, they believed, broke away and spread in the late stages of the disease, when it had overtaken the lymph nodes. New evidence not only pointed to the circulation of the blood as the means by which cancer spread but, worse, it suggested that the rogue cancer cells began to migrate to other parts of the body during the very early stages of the disease. The limitations of surgery alone as a cure for cancer became all too clear.

Radiotherapy also failed to permanently cure most cancers, although it was very effective at shrinking cancers and delaying the course of the disease. Both X-rays and gamma rays were used, the former coming from electrical machines and the latter from the degradation of radioactive materials (isotopes). Radium itself was replaced by other, less dangerous, elements, such as the isotope cobalt-60, which were actually more effective. Radioactive iodine was used, with some success, to treat cancers of the thyroid, and as early as 1922 cancer of the larynx could be cured by radiotherapy, particularly when it was discovered at an early stage. Later, radiotherapy equipment became much more advanced. The rays could be targeted on the cancer with much greater precision, and so much larger doses could be given without risk to surrounding healthy tissue. But even then, radiotherapy alone was more of a palliative treatment than a curative one for most cancers.

Major advances in cancer treatment came not until after the Second World War, and one of the keys to greater success was chemotherapy. The discovery of chemotherapy began with a tragic event. In 1943, during that second world conflict, a US army ship, the *John E. Harvey*, carrying 100 tons of nitrogen mustard – the choking and blinding mustard gas of the First World War – was bombed in an air raid on Bari harbour in Italy. Many crewmen were killed by the uncontrollable release of the toxic gas. Two American scientists, Louis Goodman and Alfred Gilman, discovered from the post-mortem examination reports of the dead that the chemical had destroyed their white lymphoid blood cells. They discovered too that the survivors of the gassing also had decreased white blood cell counts. They speculated that it was possible that nitrogen mustard could be used to treat lymphoma, a cancer involving the uncontrolled proliferation of these lymphoid cells. They were proven to be right.

A few years later, Sidney Farber, a scientist at Harvard, discovered that the vitamin folic acid was critical to the growth of malignant blood cells in a certain type of childhood leukaemia, called acute lymphoblastic leukaemia. His theory, again found to be correct, was that a chemical which destroyed or compromised folic acid, would lead to a suppression of the leukaemic cells. In the first clinical trials of both nitrogen mustard and the anti-folic acid preparation, patients with these cancers of the blood went into remission, albeit for a short period. These particular cancer-killing drugs were improved and refined, and new ones were discovered. The new medicines still temporarily suppressed rather than cured the cancers but, nevertheless, medical science had discovered that cancer cells could be destroyed by the action of antagonistic chemicals. It was a monumental breakthrough in cancer treatment.

In 1965 doctors at the National Cancer Institute in the USA went further and postulated that a combination of cancer-killing drugs, rather than just a single one, might be more effective. This was the approach to treatment that had brought about the cure of patients with tuberculosis. They experimented by using four drugs simultaneously to treat acute lymphoblastic leukaemia. The treatment was given the name MOPP after the four drugs used: nitrogen mustard, oncovin, prednisolone and procarbazine. Excitingly, they found that children treated with this combination of chemicals went into long-term remission from the disease.

Using a different combination of drugs called ABVD (standing for adriamycin, bleomycine, vinblastin and dacarbazine), other doctors found the same results for patients with lymphoma and Hodgkin's disease. Refining and improving the efficacy of these drugs further, these calamitous diseases, which previously had always been fatal, had become curable. It was a fantastic result, not least because the cancers that were now conquerable, very often occurred in children and adolescents. Combination drug therapy, moreover, opened the eyes of oncologists to the possibility of using a series of different treatments, as well as different drugs, to fight cancer.

Research indicated that chemotherapy was most effective when used to destroy smaller tumours, so there was a logic in using surgery to remove the mass of the cancer, followed by chemotherapy or radiotherapy to mop up the remaining malignant cells. Early clinical testing found that tumours of the bone could be cured if a course of methotrexate, one of the anti-folic acid drugs, was given after surgery to remove the visible cancer. This approach, called adjuvant therapy, quickly became the standard treatment for many types of cancer. The treatment of bowel cancer was made more effective by the use of the drug 5-flourouracil (known as 5FU) after surgery to remove the tumour. Paclitaxel (Taxol) made the surgical treatment of ovarian cancer more effective and, similarly, the survival of breast cancer was shown to radically improve with follow-up chemotherapy. For other patients with seemingly inoperable cancer, chemotherapy or radiotherapy could be given to shrink the size of a tumour until a surgical intervention became a practical treatment.

These advances from the late 1960s onwards certainly did not mean that most cancers had become curable. On the contrary, the early detection of the disease remained (and still remains) the most important factor in cure and survival, and cancers of the lung, breast, digestive system and prostate, and melanoma of the skin have continued to take their toll. Indeed, 160,000 or more people in Britain were dying of the disease each year throughout the late 1980s. But there were now bright patches in the sky. The advances in palliative medicine described in the last chapter meant that for many patients, whose cancer had not been discovered in time for cure to be possible, the remaining years or months of life could be managed to keep them free from pain and other symptoms. Cancer remained an appalling prospect for patient and family alike, but it no longer meant almost certain death, and even when cure was unlikely, it did not mean an agonising and helpless death.

Under Douglas Scott, Macmillan began to reflect this more positive outlook. Scott began his report for the charity's annual review of 1989–90 by saying that,

> This year 250,000 in Britain will be diagnosed as having some form of cancer. One in three of the population will contract the disease at some stage in their lives, and at any one time there will be around one million cancer patients in this country. These are the facts.

But he could qualify this gloomy picture in his next paragraph with,

> Against them, however, there are some considerably more heartening figures. Thanks to advances in treatment, one third of all those with cancer recover completely. And an increasing number of those with the disease are living far longer and enjoying more satisfying lives.

Getting this message across to the public became one of Macmillan's constant themes over the following years, but it would not be easy to change the public perception of cancer. Initiated by Susan Butler early in 1988, Macmillan conducted a survey of people's attitudes to cancer.[2] The results, which must have come as no surprise, were that people were still in great fear of the disease and utterly pessimistic about its outcome. One respondent said: 'It just eats you away and it's a lot of pain and a lot of suffering on a person who's got it and those who are left behind.' Another said: 'I don't think you could live a normal life. You go for it in the first four of five months until it gets too bad, and then that'd be you. ...' And another: 'I suppose cancer is so final. What can you say to someone who's dying? ... It's just an embarrassment.'

These attitudes to cancer had been built up over many years, indeed over many decades. The reluctance of doctors and nurses to speak of the disease, the refusal of governments to encourage greater awareness of cancer, the hair-raising reporting of cancer by the popular press, plus direct experience of the illness, had all contributed to the cancer taboo. The consequences were highly damaging. They led to untold anguish among the sick and the worried well alike. People experiencing symptoms that might be cancer were put off from seeking early medical advice for fear of hearing the worst news. Since early detection was so critical for a chance of cure, lives were without doubt being lost prematurely.[3]

They also led to feelings of utter hopelessness and despair among patients who had been diagnosed with the disease, and to similar feelings among their families and friends. People with cancer were often frightened, lonely and desolate, and their loved ones equally so.

Scott began his time with Macmillan with a new approach. The theme was 'Living with Cancer'. In contrast to the heart-rending stories of despair that had characterised many of the old Society's reports until the 1960s, much more emphasis was now given to how modern treatments and care, both curative and palliative, could help patients cope with the disease and even live very full lives. The story of Connie Cowden, published in the 1987–88 annual review, was a good example.

> [Connie] was diagnosed as having cancer in 1985, after secondary tumours were discovered in a broken rib that would not heal. After a short course of radiotherapy, [she], a senior nurse in an operating theatre, was back at work. For a year she felt better. ...
>
> Connie then got worse, then better, then worse again. In September 1987 she was admitted into the Macmillan unit in Northwood. The disease had spread to her spine and right leg and she was literally paralysed with pain.
>
> 'The people here have been absolutely marvellous,' said Connie, 'Nothing is too much trouble for them. They care so much about every one of us.
>
> 'When I first came here I was in such excruciating pain that I couldn't move at all – or even think. I don't think many people expected me to

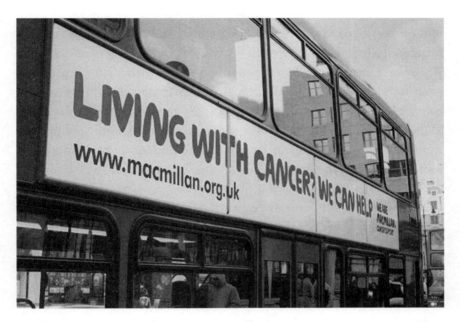

A London bus in more recent times supporting Macmillan.

survive. Now I can walk – although only for short distances, and I'm not in pain. … I know the cancer might come back. But I also know that I have already conquered it twice – against the odds. I can't pretend that having cancer doesn't make me feel a bit sorry for myself sometimes, but I believe you've always got to have goals in life. I am planning to go on holiday to Europe this year and next year I want to go to Egypt. Also, I want to do a course in bereavement counselling so that I can use the knowledge I've gained through being a nurse and having cancer to help others.'

Whether Connie made it to Europe, let alone Egypt, is not known. But what is certain is that this lady had extraordinary courage and a determination, with her doctors' help, to live her life despite the cancer. Her story must have been an inspiration and a hope to others living with cancer.

To support this much more positive message of hope, Macmillan published its first directory called *Help is There* in 1989. The publication was a list of national organisations, mostly charitable, that could provide a range of help and supportive services for people with cancer. One million copies of the booklet were printed and distributed to clinics, surgeries, libraries and Citizens Advice Bureaux UK-wide. *Help is There* was an early attempt to provide patients with a simple guide to what help could be offered, such as cancer information, counselling, befriending and practical support services, and where to go for them. Macmillan's patron, the Duchess of Kent, launched the new publication at a gathering of 200 cancer patients, some undergoing treatment and some who had been cured. These included Diana Moran, well known at the time as the BBC television fitness expert 'the Green Goddess', and Bob Champion, the famous National Hunt jockey whose successful battle against cancer had been told in the film *Champions*, released in 1984.[4] Another of the 200 patients at the launch, Sally Tunnadine, summed up the growing optimism by saying, 'The message [we were] putting across is that people should never give in. There is always hope and help at hand.'

Help is there, updated and enlarged, has been in print ever since. Its success, if measured only by the constant requests for copies, has been a part of the growing demand from patients and their families for more information about cancer and all to do with it. The silence of the pre-war and immediate postwar years would no longer do. The four associated charities supported by Macmillan had each been founded, in part, in response to this need, and *Help is There* gave details of these and many similar organisations.

There were charities and help-lines with a special interest and expertise in the leukaemias, Hodgkin's disease, brain tumours, cancers of the oesophagus, retinoblastoma (a childhood cancer of the eye), and testicular cancer. Over the years more and more have become established so that today almost every major cancer type has one or more organisations dedicated to the support of those with the condition. Perhaps the most notable manifestation of this growing hunger for more information about cancer was the success of the cancer information charity CancerBackup, founded in 1985 by Vicky Clement-Jones, a young doctor at St Bartholomew's Hospital in London. Clement-Jones was terminally ill with cancer. Reflecting on her illness and her treatment she said that she 'was struck by the great need for information that both patients and their families had. ... For the average patient and family members the diagnosis of cancer brought a bewildering and frightening world' and she wanted to 'kick cancer out of the closet'.[5]

Clement-Jones spoke for many. CancerBackup became the foremost organisation in the field, providing a telephone information and advice line, and producing a series of excellent publications about different cancers, their symptoms, treatment options and side effects. In summary, CancerBackup was endeavouring to answer any and every question that a patient with cancer or his or her family might want to ask. It was a far cry from the Trappist-like attitudes that had gone before.[6] Macmillan was eager to support these initiatives and gave financial support to CancerBackup before it ultimately merged with Macmillan in 2008 (see chapter 18). It was yet another of Douglas Macmillan's visions starting to be realised.

The more positive environment of cancer treatment led to other new and innovative Macmillan services. Predominantly, the Macmillan nurses so far appointed had been nurses working at the terminal care end of cancer care. Their special expertise was in the care of the dying patient and the dying patient's family. The emphasis now began to change, and Macmillan nurses with a broader expertise in cancer care and those with a special knowledge of different types of cancer were appointed. There were Macmillan nurses who specialised in chemotherapy, others who specialised in breast cancer, bowel cancer, cancers of the head and neck, or lymphoedema. Paediatric Macmillan nurses were appointed with a special knowledge of childhood cancers, and also Macmillan haematology nurses, with special skills to care for patients with leukaemia, myeloma and other cancers of the blood.

Many of these nurses would be able to be with their patients from the time of diagnosis, right through until the end of the illness. Their role was to support patients and their families, not just with traditional medical and nursing care and emotional support, but through providing the information patients and relatives might ask for. Patient after patient recalled being devastated or numbed when told by the doctor that they had cancer. It was, and still is, a terrifying prospect and a traumatic experience. Patients would often take little in when first given the news. The Macmillan nurse caring for the patients from the very beginning could be ready, at any time, to give to the patient the answers to the countless number of questions they would have liked to ask the doctor. The experience of Sharon Reeve, aged just 24, was recorded in 1989,

[Sharon] doesn't remember much about the day ... that doctors told her that she had non-Hodgkin's lymphoma. At that time it was just cancer ... but she doesn't forget meeting Macmillan nurse Anne Bew ...

'Anne didn't bombard me with information I couldn't absorb. She suggested we should go home and talk.'

Anne gave Sharon her telephone number and Sharon's mother admits that the phone was in constant use during the first weeks. Once the initial shock faded they had many questions to ask about the disease and its treatment.

Another story was that of Bridget Wilkinson. She was 38 when she was told she had a potentially fatal brain tumour. Well into the course of the disease she said: 'I want to know everything about each drug I take – what it is, how it controls pain, any side-effects and so on. Jeanette [her Macmillan nurse] gets all the answers. ...'

The new types of Macmillan nurse added another fillip to the Macmillan nurse programme. Rita O'Brien left Macmillan in 1988, but Scott appointed in her place the equally shrewd Loretta Tinckham, a former NHS manager who, like O'Brien, had extensive contacts throughout the regional and area health authorities that gave the go-ahead and provided the funds for new services to patients.

The Macmillan nurse programme was also aided by the appointment of regional advisers in palliative care. The regional advisers were employed by the Regional Health Authorities[7] of the NHS, but they were funded by Macmillan. Their brief was to encourage and develop better palliative care services across their region. The advisers, who were all nurses and many of them former Macmillan nurses, played an important role defining and shaping palliative care in their regions. They worked closely with O'Brien and then Tinckham, and smoothed the way for the development of new Macmillan nurse posts.[8] By 1990 nearly 800 Macmillan nurses were in place, and by the time Scott retired in 1995, there were more than 1,200. The Prince of Wales attended a celebratory lunch to mark the appointment, in 1993, of the 1,000th

Macmillan nurse. She was Rachel Ducker, a paediatric cancer specialist, based at the Leicester Royal Infirmary Children's Hospital.

Macmillan's programme of buildings also changed its emphasis. The wave of construction of continuing care units or inpatient hospices within the National Health Service had ended, as we have seen, with the cut-backs in public expenditure during the late 1970s and the shift towards care in the community. Tight public expenditure budgets within the NHS never allowed the inpatient programme to pick up again in any significant way. However, a new concept had been pioneered at St Luke's Nursing Home in Sheffield, and this was the day hospice. It was another idea from the ever-fertile and ebullient mind of Eric Wilkes. He had observed that so many patients admitted to St Luke's as inpatients could be discharged back home once their pain and other symptoms had been brought under control. The progress of their disease was manageable, so long as they had a regular review of their palliative treatment from clinicians skilled in the discipline. This medical review could take place at a day hospice.

Day care, as it came to be called, had many similarities to the services offered at day centres for the elderly or severely disabled. Apart from the clinical supervision, it could give patients a day away from home with a variety of therapies available to make them more comfortable or to lift their spirits. At the same time, it could give their carers at home a much-needed break from the daily routine of looking after their loved one. Wilkes saw the day hospice as back-up for the routine care of patients at home, most of whom should be able to stay at home until the end. He thought that the inpatient hospice should be the long stop for exceptional cases. The voluntary hospices soon followed the Sheffield lead and built new day centres attached to their inpatient units.

With this new dimension, and under the direction of Derek Spooner, the emphasis of Macmillan's building programme shifted towards the construction of these cancer day centres, or day hospices, as they were also known. The first day care centres were incorporated into the Macmillan continuing care units, either at the time of construction or later through adaptations to the building or extensions to it. Even by the time Garnett retired many of the units, including those at Oxford, Christchurch, Northampton and Nottingham, had facilities to offer day care to a dozen or more patients, and there were plans in hand for others, including Southampton and Norwich.

A new approach came with a scheme to provide a comprehensive Macmillan service in west Berkshire. The scheme was put together in partnership with the West Berkshire Health Authority, and included the construction of an inpatient unit and integrated day care centre at Dellwood Hospital in Reading, together with day centres, standing alone, at Wokingham Hospital and at Sandleford Hospital in Newbury.[9] The day centres were completed in 1990. They included consulting and treatment rooms and space for other activities, and were equipped with baths adapted for the frail or disabled, hairdressing facilities and aids to help rehabilitation. They were able to offer patients a wide range of treatments and services, including medical and nursing care, physiotherapy and complementary and occupational therapies.

The two day centres were an integral part of the support services for patients being cared for at home. Liz Ormerod, a Macmillan nurse attached to the day centre in Newbury, said:

> The day care unit is an important place for social contact for patients who are living at home, especially those who are on their own. Patients come once or twice a week, depending on their needs.

Dr Paul Millard, a local general practitioner with a special interest in palliative care, said that:

> The centre provides a way of monitoring patients' symptoms in a very friendly and relaxed environment. It's giving the best medical care whilst allowing patients to live a normal life.

Over the next few years, new standalone cancer day centres would be built in many locations, including Andover, Peterborough, Lanchester, St Albans, Ascot and Bishop Aukland, while others would be integrated into inpatient facilities. Elsewhere, Macmillan continued its support for the voluntary hospices by sponsoring fund-raising appeals for new day centres. As always, the precondition that Macmillan applied to any new building project was that the new service so created had to be a part of the local health authority's integrated plan for palliative care.

The west Berkshire project was notable for another reason. The Macmillan buildings at Reading, Newbury and Wokingham were the first to be constructed on a new design concept developed specifically for Macmillan by a firm of architects called Architects Design Partnership (ADP). The Oxford Method of building construction had served Macmillan well in the early years when the priority was to get the new services up and running as soon as possible, but it did not create buildings of internal or external aesthetic quality. This was to change. The heart of the ADP design concept was that there should be a large area in the centre of the building which would be used for the main day centre and for all communal activity. It was always a bright and airy space, and both comfortable and safe. Off this area would be the treatment and therapy rooms, consultation rooms, the adapted bathrooms, hairdressing salon, kitchens and often a small chapel. The concept was called Macmillan Green, likening the main day centre area to a communal green in the centre of a village, around which are situated all the other amenities.

The Macmillan Green design was very flexible. It could be scaled up or down to meet the projected number of patients, and it could be adapted to different shapes and sizes of land. It could also be used for inpatient continuing care units. Macmillan Green broke with the past in another way. These new Macmillan buildings were built with traditional materials and not by systems methods. This allowed for much better quality of design and finish, and much greater flexibility to meet patients' needs and patient comfort. The objective was to create Macmillan centres that really were homes from home for patients. Comfortable armchairs, carpets, fireplaces and hearths, bathrooms with patterned tiles, good quality wallpaper decoration and many other touches created an atmosphere of restful, friendly and safe domesticity. All this was a far cry from the cold, clinical and disinfected air that patients were used to in other parts of the hospital.

These new dimensions to Macmillan's work, and more would come later, added to the ever-growing demand for new Macmillan services. Figures calculated by the Cancer Research Campaign suggested that, by 1990, more than one million people would be living with cancer at any time. Scott estimated that of these sufferers, only about 60,000 would come into contact with a Macmillan service or a service from one of the associated charities. He rightly pointed out that if Macmillan could increase its services so that three times more cancer patients could benefit from them, still only one in five people with cancer would be helped. It was true that the voluntary hospices were expanding their work and coverage, and that many provided a comprehensive inpatient, day-patient and home care service. However, they were able to care for only a minority of patients – probably about 10 per cent – who were terminally ill with cancer. The vast majority of patients relied on the National Health Service for the whole of their care, and this was where Scott intended to concentrate Macmillan's future efforts.

As Scott was often to point out, 'The charity is only as good as its ability to raise money.'

Notes & References

1. In the 1990s the rate rose to one in four.
2. *Public Attitudes to and Knowledge of Cancer in the UK*, CRMF, 1988.
3. And they still are. The writer has direct knowledge of a patient with colon cancer in 2002 who, despite indicative symptoms over a long period, did not seek medical attention until the disease had spread to the liver. A cancer that might well have been curable ended with the patient's death.
4. Champion had been diagnosed with cancer in 1979, but after a year of intensive treatment he was able to ride to victory in the 1981 Grand National.
5. See *Cancer & Beyond: The formation of CancerBackup* by Vicky Clement-Jones, published in the BMJ, 12 October 1985, vol. 291, pp. 1021–3.
6. The Cancer Research Campaign also developed programmes of cancer information.
7. The National Health Service structure in England was reorganised in 1974 into fourteen regional health authorities, which planned and coordinated most health services, leaving day-to-day management to area health authorities and district management teams.

8. The voluntary hospices were wary of this development, for it increased further the influence of Macmillan within the NHS, possibly to the detriment of voluntary hospices seeking financial support for their range of services.

9. The scheme also included the refurbishment of the radiotherapy department at the Royal Berkshire Hospital in Reading.

14

The Macmillan Nurse Appeal

In 1987, Douglas Scott's first year at Macmillan, the charity had an income of £10.3 million (about £17.8 million today), and it spent on Macmillan services nearly £7.7 million. At the average rate of growth at the time, which was steady but not remarkable, Scott estimated that income could rise to about £15 million in 1991 and to £30 million at the turn of the century. This would be adequate to cover the planned growth of new Macmillan services at the current rate, although only just, but it would not allow for an expansion of those programmes. In fact, in 1995, Scott's last year at Macmillan, income had risen to a little over £39 million (about £46 million today), and spending on services £29.2 million. This growth of income, particularly during the early nineties, made Macmillan the fastest growing charity in the country.

When Scott took over the reins there was surely no disagreement about the need for Macmillan to grow. There were, however, questions about the ability of the charity to get much bigger and the suitability of its structures and governance. The first problem was a slightly technical accounting issue, but one with considerable implications. Macmillan's financial support for each new Macmillan nurse was typically for a three-year period. For a medical or university post it was more likely to be for a five-year period. In the case of Macmillan buildings, it would be for the cost of the building, but spread over the period of construction. Existing practice was that before a new Macmillan service was introduced, whether it was a Macmillan nurse or doctor, or a new Macmillan building, the full costs of the service had to be held in the charity's funds. This meant that, for example, before a new Macmillan nurse post was approved, a sum to cover the funding for the full three years had to be transferred to the charity's reserve funds. This was despite whether or not the full amount had yet been raised by the local fund-raising activities.

This was a very conservatively prudent approach. It left the charity with two options. It could hold back on the appointment of the new nurse until the full cost of the three-year commitment had been raised; although the evidence was that fund-raising was much more effective when the nurse was in post and the local charity-giving public could see what they were being asked to pay for. Moreover, these additional nurses were urgently needed, and delaying their appointment could only be to the detriment of patients and families. The alternative option was for Macmillan to regularly carry a huge reserve of general funds, sufficient to cover all of its commitments. This was an equally unattractive solution because donors are rightly suspicious of charities which hold vast sums of money in the bank, leaving aside the question of how Macmillan would build up such a bank balance in the first place.

This accounting practice did not take into account the fact that fund-raising for new Macmillan nurses, doctors and buildings often took place over two or three years. To draw an analogy from the commercial sector, it was as if a company manufacturing cars should not be able to build one unless it had been sold and paid for. As it stood, this accounting strategy was an unnecessarily cautious brake on the charity's expansion. The chairman Hugh Dundas and Douglas Scott raised this problem with the charity's auditors, the City of London firm, Dixon Wilson. The auditors understood the problem. They agreed a new formula which required that the reserves fund needed only to cover the next twelve months of expenditure, anticipating that future fund-raising would cover subsequent expenditure. This change allowed Macmillan to expand on a scale bigger then ever.

The second problem led partly from the first. Macmillan's legal structure as a benevolent society registered under the Friendly Societies Acts was not really appropriate for a rapidly growing charity which entered into commercial contracts with suppliers and into commitments of many millions of pounds. In fact, the structure had changed little since Douglas Macmillan had concluded his reorganisation of the charity to form the National Society for Cancer Relief in 1924.

The governing body was still the elected council, now of fifty people, which met four times a year. The members of the council were the charity's trustees, who were legally responsible and accountable for all that was done in the charity's name. In practice, a much smaller Finance and General Purposes Committee took many of the day-to-day decisions that were needed if the organisation was not to slow to a halt, but the council could not derogate its legal and moral obligations, even if it wanted to. Of greatest worry to anyone contemplating joining the council was that the trustees of a benevolent society were ultimately responsible, and personally so, for the affairs of the organisation. This was not a risk so long as the charity limited itself to raising funds for a programme of patient grants. But now it had grown into a multi-million pound concern, the level of attention required from the trustees had increased accordingly. Yet another problem was the somewhat archaic and increasingly inapposite law that governed friendly and benevolent societies. For example, it prevented Macmillan from investing its reserve funds in anything other than the safest of bonds, offering the lowest returns – often lower than the rate of inflation. It was beyond doubt that further expansion of Macmillan was untenable unless the charity had a new structure.

The solution, recommended by solicitor Christopher Seaman, the new secretary appointed shortly after Douglas Scott, was that the charity should convert from a friendly society to a charitable company, limited by guarantee. This was a structure increasingly favoured by charities of all sizes but particularly medium and larger-sized charities, and one which could bring the more effective accountability and flexibility that a growing charity needed. A charitable company, like its commercial counterpart, has limited liability, and so its trustees do not risk their own

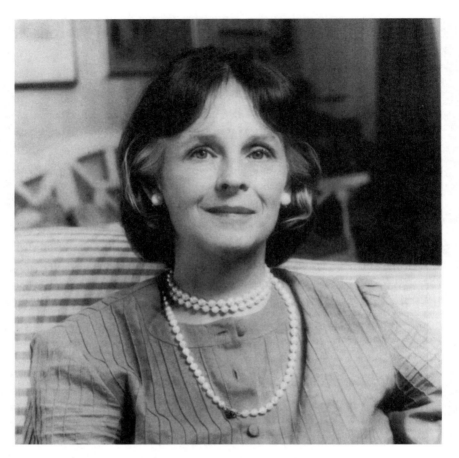

The Countess of Westmorland.

funds in the event of insolvency.[1] The charitable company's members, instead of buying shares, agree to guarantee a sum of money, usually just £1 each, in the event of an insolvency. Seaman's recommendation was put to the council in November 1988, and Dundas introduced the discussion by saying that the changes 'were intended to make the constitution fit the business, rather than make the business fit the constitution'. The council supported the proposals and agreed to call an Extraordinary General Meeting of members on 19 April 1989. The members too supported the conversion of the charity into a company limited by guarantee, and on 30 June 1989, Macmillan became an English registered company.

The trustees of the new charitable company were the members of the Finance and General Purposes Committee of the old benevolent society. They included, of course, Hugh Dundas and Richard Hambro,[2] and also the Countess of Westmorland,[3] but the opportunity was also taken to appoint new members, and particularly some with professional palliative care knowledge. One was Dr (afterwards Professor) Geoffrey Hanks, a leading physician in palliative care from the Royal Marsden Hospital. Another was Baroness McFarlane of Llandaff, Professor of Nursing at the University of Manchester. Martyn Lewis, the TV newsreader, also joined the trustees. It was, as well, time for some farewells, as Dr Ronnie Fisher and Sir Charles Davis retired after many years of quite exceptional service to the charity and, in the case of Fisher, to the dedicated care of patients as well.

The new and continuing trustees became known, collectively, as the Board, and as well as having the status of trustees, they became the directors of the charitable company. The council ceased to have any executive or decision-making powers, and was instead reconstituted as an advisory body to assist and counsel the Board. Since, unlike most large charities, Macmillan remained a members' organisation, the council was there to provide that important link and channel of communication between Board and local supporters, and particularly the voluntary fund-raising committees. With Macmillan's metamorphosis into a charitable company with robust structures, a new stage of development could be contemplated with much greater confidence.

Generating Macmillan's income had already become ever more complex and sophisticated. Across the United Kingdom, Macmillan's committees of volunteers had grown in number so that by the time of incorporation there were about 600 of them. In 1989 the committees raised about £2.8 million, or one-fifth of Macmillan's total income that year of £14 million. Given that, for the most part, fund-raised income by the committees was free from staff and other costs, it was a very valuable source of money. Another voluntary committee, called the London Events Committee, had been formed to organise prestigious and large-scale events in the capital. Chaired by an extraordinarily hardworking and enthusiastic lady called Tor Petley,[4] the committee was a great success, not only by bringing in significant funds, but also by

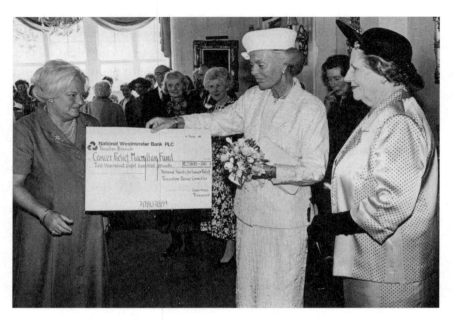

The Duchess of Kent receives a cheque from members of the Taunton Deane Committee.

further raising Macmillan's profile with important and influential groups of people. Its annual events included the 'tug of war' contest between the two Houses of Parliament, the City of London gulls' eggs lunch, the Palace of Westminster variety show, and a very grand Christmas fair. Although there is no accurate figure for the number of people who voluntarily helped to organise fund-raising events for Macmillan, the number must have been several thousand.

The programme of local appeals, as proposed by Hugh Dundas back in 1984 and led by Simon Lloyd, had proven to be a great success. As each new Macmillan nurse came into post, a local appeal for funds to pay the nurse's salary and other costs was opened in the area where the nurse would be working. Similarly, local appeals were opened to meet the costs of the new Macmillan buildings, and other larger appeals were for several nurses, or for nurses and a building.

Local appeals were an effective fund-raising vehicle because they directly linked the community of an area with its new cancer care service. People were asked to give not to a nebulous or distant cause, but towards the cost of a Macmillan service that might later benefit them, or their families or their friends. Well-known or well-respected local people would often agree to join an appeal committee, and many would make their own financial contributions so that the appeal could be launched with some exuberance. Macmillan's web of friends and contacts grew wider and wider as business leaders, councillors, churchmen, personalities and trade union officials were asked to get involved, echoing the advice about organising committees published by the old Society sixty years before. Local appeals were so successful that many of them exceeded their targets by considerable margins, leaving surpluses that could be used to pay for other local Macmillan initiatives. Interestingly, some of the appeals which closed with the biggest surpluses were from the poorest of communities. For example, an appeal for £90,000 to pay for a Macmillan nurse for the Merthyr and Cynon Valleys, very depressed mining areas of south Wales, actually raised £195,000, the balance being used to add to the number of nurses. Only one or two local appeals disappointed expectations.

Impressive as this steady growth and development was, it was not sufficient to bring about the rapid escalation of Macmillan work that Douglas Scott and his colleagues wanted to see. In 1989 Macmillan had received requests from the NHS for money to pay for another 120 Macmillan nurses to care for patients at home. The charity had the capacity only to raise funds for another forty. Estimates were that more than 400 new Macmillan nurses were needed to work with patients in NHS hospitals, and these figures did not include the need for Macmillan nurses working in paediatrics or other specialist fields. On top of this almost insatiable demand for more Macmillan nurses was the cost of providing the specialist education and training to support them. Scott estimated that in 1990 alone, there was a shortfall of some £60 million between what Macmillan could reasonably expect to raise, and what could be beneficially spent on new Macmillan nursing services. It was pretty obvious that Macmillan had to look to a very long haul before the reach of its nursing services could be anywhere near comprehensive.

The year 1991 was the 80th anniversary of the charity's beginnings with the death of Douglas Macmillan's father. Scott and Lloyd, strongly supported by Dundas, saw this as an opportunity to mount not only a new, but also a landmark national appeal for funds. Most of

Macmillan's funds came from the average man or woman who gave a few pounds each year, or from the fund-raising activities of the local committees. A new appeal could be directed at companies and grant-giving trusts which hitherto, with a few exceptions, had not been among Macmillan's greatest or most regular benefactors. Moreover, the campaign of advertising and publicity that would be needed to support and sustain a major appeal would inspire many other men and women to become regular Macmillan donors. Douglas Scott had seen that another charity, the National Society for the Prevention of Cruelty to Children (NSPCC) had launched just such a large-scale appeal, after which its yearly income from fund-raising remained on a much higher plateau, and he was determined to see Macmillan follow this example. Dundas spoke to the Council[5] about the appeal and said he was sure that 'it would have far-reaching and long-term consequences. ... It was a foundation for a vastly enhanced income for years to come.'

A leading expert in charity fund-raising at this time was Redmond Mullin, and he was consulted for his advice and expertise. He had no doubt that Macmillan's cause was a compelling one and he confirmed the figure of £15 million as a potential, although challenging, target to set. This figure could also have been regarded as, at best, overly ambitious and even fanciful. Less than ten years before, as we have seen, a national appeal for only £3 million began to wither, and was closed having achieved just two-thirds of the target. This was before the Macmillan nurse had really begun to fire the public imagination but, nevertheless, the appeal target of £15 million represented for Macmillan one whole year's income. Such an enterprising exercise required a great deal of planning and preparation, and this took up much of 1990. Brochures and leaflets had to be drafted, events planned, venues booked, additional staff taken on, and business and community leaders recruited to special committees. Susan Butler was ready to plan the advertising campaign and commission a video film for the appeal's official launch. However, one of the most important matters to be resolved was how the appeal should be directed and managed. Mullin had suggested one or two options, but identifying the leaders of the appeal was critical. Luck was on Macmillan's side.

Anthony Simonds-Gooding was a marketing and public relations executive of some distinction. He had been group managing director of Whitbread & Co., chairman and chief executive of Saatchi plc, and in 1987 he became chief executive of British Satellite Broadcasting, or BSB as it was known. In 1990 BSB was taken over by Sky Television, and Simonds-Gooding was out of a job. Meanwhile, it came to Scott's attention that Simonds-Gooding and his wife had become members of Macmillan's London Events Committee. Scott at once offered Simonds-Gooding the job of running the new appeal and, according to Scott slightly to his surprise, Simonds-Gooding accepted. Simonds-Gooding's wife Marjorie was being treated for cancer, and reflecting on his decision to take on the challenge he said: 'I was determined to do something I really wanted [to do] – and this will be a labour of love.'

There could have been no better candidate.[6] Apart from his mastery of his profession, his imaginary approach brought an exciting new component to the appeal. The appeal was given greater clarity and focus as The Macmillan Nurse Appeal, and a by-line, 'Fighting cancer with more than medicine', was added. These connected strongly with research sponsored by Macmillan showing the emotional and psychological damage brought about by a diagnosis of cancer, and the need patients had for the support of a Macmillan nurse from this early point in the process of the disease. The funds raised by the Macmillan Nurse Appeal would be used particularly to increase the number of hospital-based Macmillan nurses by 260. Simonds-Gooding was so confident about this approach that he recommended the already very ambitious appeal target be increased from £15 million to £20 million. And to give the appeal its own distinctive personality, Simonds-Gooding introduced a green, floppy bow as its logo or symbol. It was a concept almost drawn on the back of an envelope, but it was hugely successful. This cheerful, bouncing, and rather idiosyncratic, image caught exactly the energy and the extrovert character of the appeal. It appeared on every single thing associated with the appeal, and it remained the charity's well-known fund-raising emblem for several years.

More luck came Macmillan's way when the Prince of Wales, responding with enthusiasm to a plea from the Countess of Westmorland, agreed to become the patron of the appeal. Like his great-great-grandfather King Edward VII, the prince had long had an interest in cancer and its treatment and care. His work for the appeal was important. He held

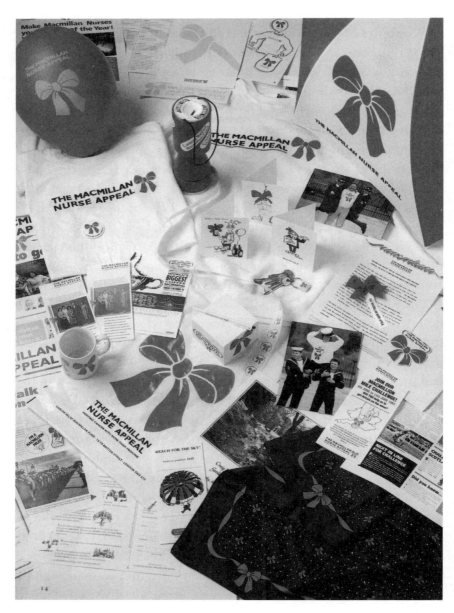

The Macmillan Nurse Appeal.

and attended receptions in support of the appeal, including one at Highgrove House, his home in Gloucestershire. The prince also made a point of visiting cancer patients in many of the hospitals where the new Macmillan nurses were to be based. His Macmillan itinerary included Glasgow and Fort William, Bristol and Boston, Gloucester and the Clatterbridge cancer hospital near Liverpool. One other piece of good luck was the decision of the 663rd Lord Mayor of London, Sir Alexander Graham, to make Macmillan the chosen charity of his 1990/1 mayoral year. As a direct result, Macmillan and its work became much better known throughout the Square Mile in the run-up to the launch of the appeal, and the charity was able to have its own float showing the work of the Macmillan nurses in the 1990 Lord Mayor's Parade.[7]

The formal and public launch of the Macmillan Nurse Appeal was on 25 September 1991. Simultaneous events were held in London, Birmingham, Manchester and Glasgow. The London launch was hosted by the prince at a reception at St James's Palace. Its theme was the feeling of despair and isolation that patients experience when told that they have cancer, and the role that Macmillan nurses based in hospitals can have in supporting these patients. The prince explained that:

> I agreed to become patron of this appeal for the simple reason that I deeply admire the labour of love carried out by these exceptional nurses and I value, above all, their selfless devotion to the care of those with cancer and their families.
>
> Like most of us I have known several people with cancer ... and they have told stories how friends avoided them, literally passed over on the other side of the street, or relatives locked in a conspiracy of silence, unable to speak openly about it.
>
> So at the very time that the person with cancer needs the most help, the people they normally depend on can leave them isolated.
>
> It is surprising ... that it isn't just friends and relatives who find it difficult to cope with, but also the very health professionals that cancer patients turn to for help and advice. They have in the past been trained to treat the disease, rather than the individual who has it. There may be reluctance to become involved with the emotional needs of patients, knowing this will demand time and counselling – skills which they don't

have. They may hide their own anxiety behind professional detachment which, to the patients, may make them appear cold and uncaring.

The prince neatly summarised the inadequacy of the care that so many cancer patients had experienced, and it was a powerful case to support Macmillan's new appeal. A video film with stories from patients, and including the words from the prince, was produced and widely distributed.

The Macmillan appeal gave vent to a burgeoning of new fund-raising ideas, and it made Macmillan one of the most innovative and vivacious of charities. Seymour Thistlethwaite, a former Greenjacket and businessman in Arabia with an acute salesman's nose, became head of corporate fund-raising, with a brief to persuade major companies to get involved with the appeal. Such a post in the charity sector at the time was most unusual and indeed it might have been unique. Thistlethwaite recruited a good team around him and, more so than anyone else, developed the concept of the 'charity of the year'.

It was not a good time for charities to ask companies for money. In 1990 the economy had started to slip into recession and business confidence had fallen dramatically. Indeed, despite all the very persuasive attempts of Dundas, it had proved impossible to find a big, business leader to become the chairman of the appeal because, so Dundas believed, they were all too taken up with the financial plight of their own companies.[8] The economy remained at a low ebb throughout the period of the appeal. Thistlethwaite and his team, not to forget Simonds-Gooding, realised that to get support from companies, Macmillan had to give something back and to be valuable to them. This could be the public association the company could have with the Macmillan name,[9] or it could be the chance for the company's staff to become involved with the charity's work. Or companies could sponsor some major fund-raising event or series of fund-raising events, and earn good publicity and public goodwill. Another option was cause-related marketing, where the charity received a small percentage of the turnover or profit made on sales.

The list of companies that supported the Macmillan Nurse Appeal was impressive. It included the Nationwide Building Society; the high street chain Next; the largest bank in the world, JP Morgan; Vauxhall Motors; and supermarkets Asda and Kwik Save. In several cases the companies retained their association with Macmillan for several years.

Just as much attention was given to raising funds from the major grant-giving trusts and charitable foundations, with which Macmillan had not been particularly successful in the past. Edward Hay, an ex-guards officer turned businessman, and with a network of highly placed contacts, was taken on to reach deeper into this sector. With close support from Hugh Dundas, in the year 1992 a total of £2.7 million was donated to the appeal by trusts and foundations, including gifts from Smith's Charity, the Wolfson Foundation, the Monument Trust and several others. Other very well-known organisations, and with quite different characteristics, supported the appeal. The Freemason's Grand Charity gave a significant sum, and help came from the WRVS. The National Garden Scheme, which had first organised the opening of private gardens to raise funds for district nurses in 1927, made the Macmillan nurses its major beneficiary. With 2,700 gardens in the scheme, this support was of enormous potential. The Club and Institute Union, or CIU, the umbrella body of the hundreds of working men's clubs in England and Wales, made Macmillan its special charity of the year and encouraged its member clubs to contribute to the cause. Finally, Helping Hands Gift Shops, a chain of over seventy charity shops located throughout England, covenanted the greater part of its profits to Macmillan.[10]

No charity appeal, particularly in modern times, will reach its potential unless it can draw in the enthusiasm and the participation of the general public. Since the appeal was intended to raise Macmillan's profile, and to push the charity permanently onto a higher plateau, a good deal of publicity, promotion and hype was required. The launch of the appeal had attracted a great deal of television and press coverage, and Susan Butler and her team ensured that this was kept going. Macmillan had long used celebrities to champion its cause with extra colour and interest, and the Macmillan Nurse Appeal was an ideal enterprise for this. The list of well-known people who gave freely of their time included the Olympic Gold swimmer Duncan Goodhew, test cricketer David Gower, Liverpool singer Gerry Marsden, wacky TV presenter

Chris Evans, and the entertainer Roy Castle.[11] Their support was particularly useful in raising interest in the two national events that had been devised for widespread public participation: the World's Biggest Coffee Morning and the Macmillion Mile Challenge.

Jill Phillips had been an actress before joining Macmillan as manager of its national fund-raising events.[12] Her greatest achievement in that role was to create the annual World's Biggest Coffee Morning. The first was launched in 1991 with sponsorship from the food company Lyons Tetley. The idea was simple. On a given morning, people all around the country, whether at home or at work, were asked to organise a coffee break for family, friends or colleagues and to ask them to donate to the Macmillan appeal. Organised coffee mornings were held by Macmillan's committees, by employees of companies which had chosen Macmillan as their 'charity of the year', by cadets at the Royal Naval College in Dartmouth, in hospitals and hospices, in government offices, in shopping malls, and even in Brixton Prison. It was estimated that over 300,000 people took part, earning the event a place in the Guinness Book of Records[13] and raising for the appeal over £250,000. In its second year, 4,700 coffee mornings were registered and together they raised nearly £500,000. The event continues to this day, growing every year.

The Macmillion Mile was another event for all to join in. Supporters could walk or run, be pushed, walk backwards, skip, or in any other way travel a mile and raise funds for the appeal. One of the more interesting miles walked, although one of rather doubtful salubriousness, was through the underground sewers of Brighton. Liz McColgan, the medal-winning runner of the Olympic and Commonwealth Games, agreed to be the patron of the event. She had lost several members of her family to cancer and reasoned that, 'There are so many people who have had the heartbreak of losing loved ones through cancer, and anything I can do to … help ease the burden of suffering … is worthwhile.'

In 1992 around 390,000 people made their imperial journey and raised £434,000. Apart from McColgan, probably the best-known Macmillion miler, and one who found the challenge no more than a piece of cake, was Desert Orchid, winner of the 1989 Cheltenham Gold Cup.

It was not just the British public that gave generously to the appeal. London has long been the home of many US citizens who work in

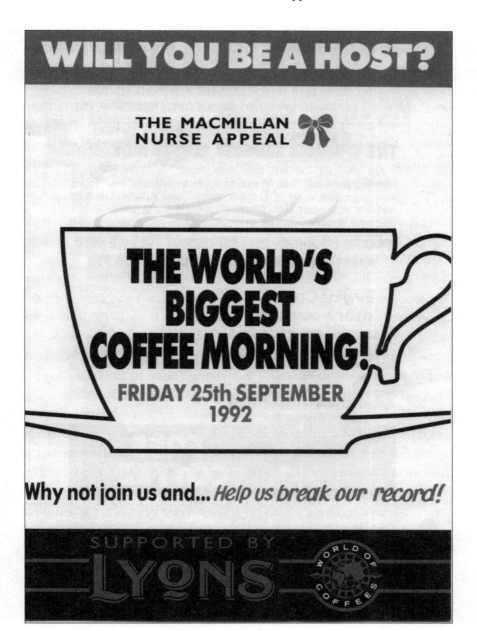

The World's Biggest Coffee Morning, 1992.

the American banks, law firms and US corporations that have offices in the capital. Many stay with their families in London for several years and play a very active part in the life of the city. A few American lawyers based in London set up an Illinois-registered US charity, now called the American Friends of Macmillan Cancer Support. As an American charity, US citizens could benefit from tax relief on their donations, and this of course made giving a much easier and more attractive thing to do.[14] The American Friends charity made many grants to Macmillan, particularly to help fund Macmillan nurses working at the London Clinic and other hospitals where American citizens living in London would be most likely to go if they were in need of medical or surgical treatment.

The Macmillan Nurse Appeal reached its target less than two years after its public launch in 1991. There can be no doubt that it was a considerable achievement, which had not only the short-term, but also the long-term impact that was intended. *Charity Trends*, published by the Charities Aid Foundation, an umbrella organisation supporting all charities, reported that Macmillan's achievement was 'striking', coming, as it did, despite a period of continuous economic recession. Between 1990 and 1995, Macmillan's income grew, on average, by nearly 25 per cent each year and it propelled Macmillan up the league of charities by size, overtaking several that were household names. By 1995 it was the tenth largest charity in terms of voluntary income. In the same period, spending on Macmillan services for people with cancer increased from £14 million to more than £29 million. There were now in post more than 1,200 Macmillan nurses, 129 Macmillan doctors and over £4 million each year was being spent on grants to patients in financial need. A rough and ready estimate suggested that about 200,000 people in 1995 were helped by one or other Macmillan services. This was three times more than Scott's estimate of the number helped just five years before.

Notes & References

1. On the other hand, they do retain personal liability for breaches of trust. It is usual today to cover this risk by insurance.

2. Hugh Dundas retired from the Board in June 1991, and was succeeded as chairman by Richard Hambro. Hambro was succeeded, in turn, as treasurer by Dundas's son, Jamie. Ten years later, Jamie Dundas was elected as chairman.

3. The countess stood down in 1990 and was succeeded as president by the Marchioness of Zetland.

4. Mrs Roderick Petley was later awarded the MBE for her charity work.

5. On 8 November 1989.

6. Simonds-Gooding undertook this role without payment. In 1992 he was elected a trustee of Macmillan, a post he held until 2001.

7. Not to be outdone, the Lord Mayor of Westminster, Dr Cyril Nemeth, chose the Macmillan appeal as beneficiary to receive all proceeds of his New Year's Day Parade in 1992.

8. The result was that Dundas himself, with the help of Richard Hambro, undertook this role.

9. The concept of a charity having its own valuable brand was just beginning to be discussed.

10. In 1994 the directors of Helping Hands Gift Shops offered to transfer the ownership of the chain to Macmillan without cost. Since many of the shops were only marginally profitable, Macmillan declined the offer. The offer was then made to the Marie Curie Memorial Foundation, which accepted. Irrespective of the financial advantages and disadvantages of the offer, it provided the Marie Curie charity with a prominent and visible advertisement in many cities and towns.

11. Castle, although never a smoker, was diagnosed with lung cancer in 1992. He believed he was the victim of inhaling the tobacco smoke of others in the clubs where he entertained. He died two years later at the age of 62.

12. Phillips was well supported by an assistant called Sophie Rees-Jones, who went on to marry Prince Edward and became the Countess of Wessex.

13. And it continued to hold its place in the Guinness Book of Records.

14. Similar tax relief was given to British tax-payers, but not until 1998.

15

Onwards and Upwards

As the Macmillan Nurse Appeal propelled the charity along, its growing size, strength and confidence meant that it could broaden its scope and look ahead. Macmillan's existing services were improved and developed, and new services were conceived and introduced. The charity also embarked on a limited overseas programme. The spirit for the following few years was raised at a two-day European conference on palliative care held in London on 12 November 1992. The conference, called *Palliative Care for All*, was sponsored by Macmillan and the Department of Health, and opened by the Prince of Wales. Its purpose was to keep the needs of people with cancer at the top of the agenda, not only of the National Health Service in Britain, but of government health agencies across Europe. The keynote speech came from Dr Jan Stjernsward, the head of the cancer and palliative care programmes of the World Health Organisation, who spoke of the growing global incidence and impact of cancer; other speakers, from Switzerland, Spain, Italy, Sweden and France, described developments in their home countries. A much-repeated theme was how cancer and palliative care had to develop to meet the needs of patients and their families in the next century.

As far as the United Kingdom was concerned the conference could not have been more timely, since the National Health Service was emerging from yet another of its reorganisations. This one, led by Health Secretary Kenneth Clarke and his successor William Waldegrave, had made really fundamental changes to the way health services were planned and commissioned. In 1989 Clarke had published a White Paper called *Working for Patients*. The heart of the proposals was the plan to split the National Health Service between *purchasers* and *providers* of health care.

Previously, the NHS health authorities had been responsible both for planning the range of health services that would be available, and for managing the hospitals and clinics that provided them. For the future, it was proposed that the health authorities would be responsible only for commissioning, or *purchasing*, health services on behalf of their local populations. Hospitals and community-based health services would become self-managing *providers* of health care, later to be called NHS trusts, operating the health services purchased by the health authorities. In addition, Clarke encouraged general practitioners also to become *purchasers*, and those that did were to be called fund-holders. The logic behind the changes was that a more efficient health service would be created, since the health authorities and fund-holding general practitioners would purchase the most cost-effective services from competing NHS trusts. An internal market within the NHS would thereby be created.

Freeing the health authorities from managing health services also meant that they could no longer be influenced by powerful practitioners operating at hospital level. Clarke argued that under his proposals, patients would be given more choice since NHS money would 'follow the patient'. The government pushed through these plans despite a great deal of opposition from within the NHS. The changes were encompassed in the National Health Service and Community Care Act 1990, and the split between *purchasers* and *providers* became effective the following year. Although the full implementation of the Act slowed a little, the Secretary of State for Health appointed in 1992, Virginia Bottomley, was clear in her determination to continue with the strategy. A former social worker, she had criticised the NHS for being monolithic and for its over-emphasis on central planning. She believed that devolved decision-making would create more dynamic and patient-orientated services.[1] Two years on, Bottomley brought in further changes, slimming down the NHS bureaucracy at regional level and at its headquarters in Leeds.

These changes in the National Health Service would inevitably have much importance for the way Macmillan worked with the NHS. In particular, it was questionable whether Macmillan's existing links into the NHS were right for the future development of new Macmillan patient services. The advisers in palliative care working for the regional health authorities, who had been funded by Macmillan just a few years before, were of less relevance in a decentralised and localised National Health Service where the power and influence of the regional health authorities had been drastically reduced. At the same time, Macmillan's links with the new hospitals and community services NHS trusts would be only half of the story, because as providers of patient services only, they could not give long-term commitments to keep Macmillan services going after the charity's initial funding had run out. Instead, Macmillan would have to work with both the new purchasers and providers, obtaining long-term commitments from the former, for Macmillan services based at the latter. This would be a major undertaking, requiring good intelligence, good contacts and flexibility. Importantly, Macmillan needed a mode of operation that could be every bit as responsive as the newly structured NHS was supposed to be innovative.

Douglas Scott was acutely aware of these problems. Macmillan's structure was already overburdened by the growing volume of work, and he could see that just adding new members of staff to the charity's head office would merely increase bureaucracy. On the contrary, he wanted Macmillan to reflect the new NHS structure and decentralise. In 1993 Scott produced his scheme to split Macmillan's organisation into five. There would be four regions covering England and Wales, and a fifth area to include Scotland and Northern Ireland. Each new area would be headed by an executive director who, Scott envisaged, would be sufficiently senior to be able to negotiate directly with the chiefs of the new NHS purchaser and provider bodies.

Macmillan's new structure became effective in January 1994, with three existing senior members of staff – Catherine Duthie, Loretta Tinckham and Keith Holmes – taking on director posts, and with two new directors – Diane Cresswell and Anthony Luke – appointed from outside. According to Scott, this structure would 'give the organisation strength at local level, and enable [it] to be more sensitive to local need'. Certainly Scott encouraged his directors to develop new services, innovative solutions and better ways of working. His primary concern was not to follow an exact blueprint of Macmillan services for the United Kingdom, which in the newly fragmented NHS might or might not be achievable. Rather, it was to ensure that the organisation was ever pushing onwards in its work, improving cancer care whenever and wherever possible, and flexible enough to take advantage of local circumstances and of local opportunities that came up. Scott believed that this would be the way to the greatest success.[2]

Scott pushed forward with several new ideas himself. He knew that the number of new Macmillan nurse posts agreed each year would begin to decline in the late 1990s, and he wanted to have available a range of new services, or 'products' as he liked to call them, making the analogy with commercial business. In 1992 Macmillan commissioned another survey, this one from the polling company MORI, and this time investigating the needs of people with cancer that were not being met by the health and social services. The survey asked the opinion of both patients and their carers, and it revealed that frequently the most glaring gap was not in medical or nursing care, but in day-to-day practical support. Patients often needed help with the housework or with shopping, with walking the dog or with looking after children. Coping with cancer was hard enough, but for many patients it was made even more difficult because of the lack of this rather obvious, and even mundane, assistance. The problem was surely not a new one. The records of patients who had, in the past, received Macmillan grants had described the problem many times before the spread of the welfare state. Although home help services offered by local authority social services departments had done something to alleviate the problem, they had never been adequate, and fifteen or more years of tightening controls of public expenditure had drastically restricted their availability.

The Countess of Westmorland had been one of the first to recognise the problem, drawing on her long experience in social work. Scott conceived a new Macmillan product that would fill this substantial gap in patient services. It was the Macmillan carer. Macmillan carers would be ready to help patients at home and their families with many everyday chores or tasks. As a domiciliary service, the carers would complement Macmillan nurses working with patients at home, and help to provide the comprehensive range of services that patients needed. Scott's logic was that the greater the support that could be offered at home, the more possible it became for patients to remain at home throughout their illness. This was the same reasoning that had driven forward the Macmillan nurse programme and, in theoretical terms at least, was equally in tune with the government's policy of encouraging more care in the community.

Scott asked his operational directors to prepare plans for Macmillan carer services in several parts of the country during 1993, and the first schemes were tested in Bath, Cheltenham and Aylesbury. This coincided with news that the Department of Health had funds in hand that could be allocated to supporting new and experimental services. Neville Teller, a former civil servant in the Department of Health and now Macmillan's Director of Operations, prepared a bid for a portion of this fund to enable several schemes to be formally established. He argued that Macmillan carers would be able to

> provide essential support for the practical care necessary to enable cancer patients to return home after treatment and to remain in their own homes; support patients, their families and their carers at the critical stages of the disease and aid a return to normal life; and be instrumental in avoiding late admissions to the acute wards in the last 48 hours of life.[3]

Teller asked for money to set up ten new carer services, each employing between six and ten Macmillan carers. He estimated that each Macmillan carer would cost about £13,000 per year to maintain, including costs of salary, travel and, importantly, training. To the Department of Health he proposed that Macmillan would finance the second year of operation, if the department would put up the money for the first. After the two years of operation he proposed that the services should be reviewed. The department agreed to the scheme, and in due course Macmillan carer services were set up in several areas, including Stockport, Wakefield, Norwich and Solihull. Within two years, nine services had been established in England and a further two in Scotland.

Although from the evidence of these pilot projects the Macmillan carer was a very useful addition to the range of services that could be offered to the cancer patient at home, the Macmillan carer did not catch the imagination in the same way that the Macmillan nurse had. There were early concerns that the role of the carer was not sufficiently defined, and that many were asked to carry out the duties of nurse auxiliaries or care assistants for which they were not trained.[4] There were also problems arising from the Macmillan carers' line management and conditions of service. However, the fundamental problem that prevented a wide-scale expansion of the service was the lack of long-term commitments from the public authorities to maintain the services in the future. Despite the intention that the Macmillan carer would help patients to remain at home with their illness rather than be forced back into hospital, the carers were a social rather than a health service. So long as Macmillan planned to remain a pump-priming organisation, this meant that the long-term financial support for carers had to come, in whole or in part, from the social services departments of local authorities, and not from the NHS.

Local authorities had already been required to take on much wider responsibility with the government's programme of community care. Aimed primarily at mental health, former hospital patients were being discharged into the community where social services departments would have to maintain a range of hostels and other support services. Although additional government funds had been transferred to local authorities to help them to meet this new challenge, there was little local government money left over to pay for Macmillan carer schemes. Without that major commitment of public funds that had fuelled the nationwide institutionalisation of the Macmillan nurse, the Macmillan carer could not be in a similar league. A few carer schemes were later set up, some of them using volunteers, and others being better described as befriending services. Some were set up in collaboration with other charities, such as Crossroads. Macmillan adopted a very flexible approach, but a large-scale expansion of Macmillan carer services remained elusive. However, the number of schemes did increase gradually, as social services authorities came to recognise the value of them.

Another of Scott's initiatives was a renewed programme of Macmillan cancer information. The charity had rather dropped out of this area of work with the retirement of Douglas Macmillan. However, as described in chapter 13, interest grew again with the 1988 Macmillan survey of attitudes to cancer and the pioneering work of CancerBackup. The public demand for more information about cancer was growing steadily. In 1992 Scott had met Maureen Newton, a former Macmillan nurse in Liverpool, who had quite determined ideas about how cancer information could better be spread. She believed, probably rightly, that many patients and their families remained very fearful of cancer and everything to do with it, and she understood the reluctance of many patients to discuss these things with their doctors. On the other hand, it was so important for people to know more about cancer if it was ever going to be conquered.

Newton's idea was to open a cancer information centre in the heart of Liverpool's main shopping area. She thought that people would be much more inclined to seek the information about cancer they wanted if they could do so away from the hospital or the doctor's surgery. A high street location was not only convenient for people; it was ordinary, familiar and as far away as possible from being clinical. In due course, shop premises were found in Ranelagh Street, in the city centre and close to the main shopping precincts, and the Macmillan Cancer Information Centre was opened for business in June 1994. The official opening was performed by actors and actresses from *Brookside*, a well-known Liverpool-based television soap opera of the time, which was featuring a storyline about one of its characters and breast cancer. A year later, the centre was visited by Dr Kenneth Calman, the Chief Medical Officer for England.

A much smaller Macmillan Cancer Information and Support Centre was opened a little later at Cinderford in Gloucestershire. The Liverpool centre was open for nearly three years, during which time it gave information and advice to many people, not just from Liverpool, but from the whole of Merseyside and beyond. It offered information

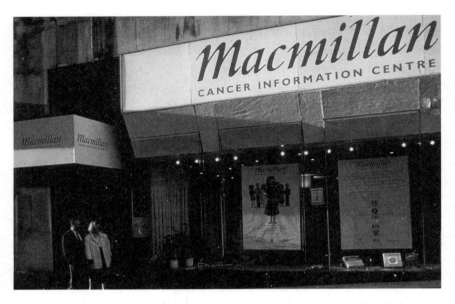

Macmillan information centre in Liverpool opened in 1994 by the stars of *Brookside*.

about the different types of cancer, their symptoms and their treatments, and about the range of medical, social and support services that were available for patients and families in the area. What was so noteworthy was how ill-informed many people were about cancer, and even about their own illness. The notion that cancer could be catching was a fear still held by some. Others thought that cancer was a certain 'death sentence' and that no treatments were effective. One patient with myeloma, a cancer of the bone marrow, thought he had the similar sounding melanoma, a skin cancer, a very different disease with quite different symptoms and treatments.

Maureen Newton reported several cases of people who had sought information from the centre about their own symptoms because they were too afraid to ask their GPs. Newton tried to persuade them to see their own doctors, even offering to go to the surgery with them. Yet other people with cancer had no idea of the social security benefits that might be available to help them and their families. The cost of operating a large high street facility was high, and without a commitment from the local NHS to make some contribution it was not feasible to maintain the centre long term. Some years later, however, a mobile

Macmillan information service was introduced, which enabled the same information and advice to be provided, but across a much bigger area.

Another new initiative to give direct help and advice to patients was the launch in April 1993 of the MAC helpline for young people with cancer aged between 13 and 20. Happily, cancer in the young is rare but, nevertheless, every year about 700 teenagers are diagnosed with some form of the disease. Cancer at any age is a traumatic experience, but for these young people it can be utterly devastating. They are already coping with all that is associated with growing up; they are thinking about schools and examinations and jobs, girlfriends or boyfriends, and on top of this turmoil comes the news of a potentially fatal illness. Treatment can mean long absences from school and friends, disability and hair loss, and the need to cope with distressed parents and siblings. At the same time, there are few hospital facilities dedicated to people in this age group, so treatment is often given on paediatric wards, alongside toddlers, or on adult oncology wards with patients who are quite elderly. Both places are quite unsuitable for adolescents. The MAC helpline was opened by the TV presenter Chris Evans and was there to offer help, support and advice on any aspect of teenage cancer and how to cope with it. It also had direct links to counselling services. Although directed chiefly at patients, the helpline also responded to calls from parents, brothers and sisters and friends.

There was much scope as well for building on existing work programmes, particularly in the field of education and training. Jennifer Raiman, the Medical Services Adviser, had been giving some priority to supporting GPs ever since the production of the MACPAC series. The role of family doctors was absolutely crucial for the better care of cancer patients. Not only were GPs responsible for much of a patient's medical care at home, they were also responsible for any referrals on to a cancer or a palliative care specialist at the local hospital or hospice. In short, a diagnostic decision of a GP about the nature of a particular symptom could have an important, and even critical, impact on the well-being of the patient. Yet, as Dr David Percy had recognised more than ten years before, most family doctors did not come across that many cancers in a year, and rare cancers they might see just once in many years of practice.

In collaboration with the Royal College of General Practitioners, Raiman developed a scheme to appoint Macmillan general practitioners, whose role was to bring GP practices closer to their local hospices and other palliative care services including Macmillan nurses, hospital oncology and radiotherapy departments, social services departments and other agencies. One of the first Macmillan GPs appointed was Dr David Butler, who worked at the Wendover Health Centre in Buckinghamshire. Talking about his work he said:

> I see myself as a facilitator, whose primary role is to help increase awareness among GPs of the different aspects of palliative care. I do this by visiting other GP practices ... to talk to doctors ... about palliative care and by running more formal training courses. ...
>
> Feedback from GPs ... shows that they are particularly interested in learning more about controlling physical symptoms, pain relief and how best to communicate with patients and their families.

Much in the spirit of Butler's description of his work, the posts were soon renamed Macmillan GP facilitators. Initially five posts were established in England and Wales, but this number rose to twenty-two by the end of 1995.

While Scott was keen to establish brand new Macmillan services, he also paid much attention to expanding and improving the existing range. Macmillan's building programme had steadily grown with the introduction of the Macmillan Green design, and its focus was now on the construction of palliative care or hospice day centres. Derek Spooner had led the development of Macmillan buildings of high quality, but the costs of construction were always rising. Scott conceived the idea of an architectural competition to test if good designs could still be produced, but at a lower cost. He approached The Prince of Wales's Institute of Architecture for help, and together, the institute and Macmillan initiated the 1992 Macmillan Design Challenge. The challenge to architects entering the competition was to design and construct a cancer day centre at lower cost, but one which would still provide the homely atmosphere and all the facilities patients needed for their treatment and care. Scott said that a Macmillan cancer day centre had to 'raise the spirit of the depressed, calm the worries of the fearful, be welcoming to those who feel isolated and give joy, and even bring humour, to those who are unhappy'. But Scott was sharp enough to recognise that 'this is a tall order for any designer'.

Twenty-six architects, or teams of architects, were admitted to the competition, and the entries were all of high quality, some of them with very innovative features intended to keep costs down. The prizes were presented by the Prince of Wales at a special ceremony at his institute. Several of the entries received a special commendation from the judges, but the winner was a young architect from Newcastle-upon-Tyne named Ian Clarke. His patient-centred, and in many ways traditional, design was later used to build the Butterwick Hospice in the grounds of the general hospital at Stockton-on-Tees. Interestingly, the competition revealed that in terms of their design and construction, Macmillan buildings were already quite cost effective.

There was one last, but important, area of activity that grew during these years, and this was Macmillan's international work. Cancer's reach was worldwide, and its impact was growing across the world, just as it had grown in the UK throughout the twentieth century. A study by the World Health Organisation of 1985 death statistics revealed that 10 per cent of all deaths were from cancer, and that the figure would grow rapidly over the forthcoming decades. Moreover, the growth would be due not to a higher incidence of cancer in the developed world, but to a huge expansion in the poorest countries of the world. It was a sad fact that most patients with cancer in the third world, where treatment facilities were inadequate, would have terminal disease. Since the foundations of hospice and palliative care were laid in the United Kingdom, it was never a surprise that doctors, nurses and health service managers from overseas would look to this country for advice, guidance and leadership. St Christopher's Hospice quite regularly held international hospice conferences and, together with several other teaching hospices, it welcomed foreign visitors on its courses or within fellowship schemes. As the success of the Macmillan nurses and other Macmillan services became more apparent and more widely known, more and more practitioners from other countries asked to visit and study Macmillan's work, and to meet the charity's senior members of staff. Given the nature of Macmillan nursing, the former was not really feasible, and the latter was very time consuming.

The first Macmillan international projects came out of the Macmillan Nurse Appeal. Sir John and Sir Adrian Swire were prominent businessmen with interests in Hong Kong, including the airline Cathay Pacific. They had agreed to generously support the appeal, but asked in return that Macmillan put on a programme of training to improve palliative care in what was then a British colony. The first course was held in 1992. In a similar vein, the Jewish community in Britain was encouraged to support the appeal and a Macmillan palliative nurse training programme was provided at the Royal Marsden Hospital for a number of Israeli nurses. This was followed by a request to organise a programme for practitioners in South Africa, and one from the Hong Kong government for a programme of advice and support. Most ambitious of all was a project to train a sufficient number of doctors and nurses in India for palliative care to be spread across the whole of the sub-continent. All in all, the programme was large enough for Tony Berry, the Patient Welfare Manager, to be given specific responsibility for it, together with the title International Manager.[5] It was always Macmillan's practice to raise specific funds to support the international projects, and mainly these would come from people with a particular link with, or interest in, the country concerned.

Douglas Scott's view[6] was that the international programme was important for several reasons. Crucially, he believed that Macmillan was 'the most suitable organisation in the world at the … time, with the experience and access to know-how, to make a major impact on the cancer care problems of the developing world', and that it 'should not turn its back on these problems'.

It was true palliative care in the community, about which Macmillan had a particular expertise, was the only realistic way of bringing relief to the millions of people in the third world who had, or who would get, the disease. However, the task of making a major impact was of truly awesome magnitude, and even the very limited overseas programme under way had been quite burdensome on Macmillan's limited staff. Scott proposed instead that Macmillan should lead and support a new international cancer care charity to take responsibility for the enormous job that would have to be done. Macmillan's Board was certainly sympathetic to the growing problem of cancer in the third world, but it did not see how Macmillan alone could lead the solutions, many of which were rooted in third world poverty as much as cancer.

Concerned about the focus of Macmillan shifting away from improving cancer services in the United Kingdom, Macmillan's overseas programme commitments were completed, but not renewed. Nevertheless, Scott kept his interest in international work, and in retirement he became trustee of an international cancer relief charity.

Notes & References

1. In fact, an effective internal market proved to be a very difficult thing to achieve, partly because of the long-term relationships that already existed between NHS staff now working for purchaser and provider bodies.
2. Introducing this programme of decentralisation within Macmillan was not without its problems, mostly caused by demarcation disputes between nationally based and regionally based directors and staff. Solutions to these problems were elusive because NHS structures and NHS policy continued to change, sometimes radically.
3. Cancer Relief Macmillan Fund Bid for DoH Support, 1993/4, prepared by Director of Operations, 10 February 1994.
4. *Evaluation of Macmillan Carer Schemes in England: Interim Report and Discussion Points*, December 1996, by Trent Palliative Care Centre and University of Sheffield.
5. A retired army brigadier and Falklands war veteran, Berry later became Director of Operations, and later still Director of Planning & Policy.
6. Writer's interview with Scott on 9 June 2005.

16

Relationships

Throughout the 1980s and 1990s Macmillan held a central, and in many ways a pivotal, role in cancer and palliative care. It worked with the Department of Health and with every level of authority within the National Health Service in almost every part of the country. It worked with the scores of voluntary hospices that had been established both before and in the wake of Cicely Saunder's founding of St Christopher's. It worked with its associated charities and with other organisations offering support and advice to patients. Finally, it worked, albeit far less closely, with the cancer research charities. No other charity in the cancer and palliative care sector had operational tentacles that were as wide or as deep. Relationships with other organisations were always crucial to Macmillan's success. The growing strength and influence of Macmillan inevitably affected these working relationships, presented dilemmas, and at times strained some of them.

The Macmillan nurse had become the charity's icon before the launch of the Macmillan Nurse Appeal. The impact of the appeal was to re-enforce that image in the public mind over and over again. Indeed, the Macmillan nurse was much more recognisable in the public mind than the charity called Cancer Relief Macmillan Fund. Cheques from donors were written in favour of *The Macmillan Nurses*, legacies were left to Macmillan nurse teams in one town or another, and requests for Macmillan nurses to speak at fund-raising events grew and grew. Many companies, trusts and other organisations, keen to support the charity, preferred to do so by sponsoring one or more Macmillan nurse, and preferably one who would work in the towns where they were based, or where they traded or operated. A good example was the very lucrative link-up between Macmillan and the *Candis Club* Magazine a little after the Macmillan Nurse Appeal had come to a close. The *Candis Club* donated several million pounds to Macmillan over three or four years, all of which was earmarked to pay for new Macmillan nurses. The Macmillan nurse was not only a skilled, professional health care worker, held so highly in the public's esteem, but also a very valuable fund-raising commodity. This predominance of the Macmillan nurse, hugely advantageous as it was, would also lead to some friction between Macmillan and its friends.

Macmillan's modus operandi from Garnett's time onwards was based on two basic tenets. First, it always collaborated with the NHS if it was at all possible, and it usually was. Second, it worked by making grants to others, again usually the NHS, in order to pump-prime new Macmillan services. It did not directly operate or manage Macmillan services (apart from the programme of welfare grants to patients) and neither did it guarantee funding for more than a fixed number of years, usually three for a Macmillan nurse. However, in return for Macmillan's funding, the operator of the new Macmillan service had agreed to maintain the service in the long term, and it also had agreed to retain the Macmillan name permanently. One observer[1] likened Macmillan's way of working to 'a very successful franchise operation'.

This approach meant that Macmillan could be very flexible and very light of foot. It also gave the charity a unique advantage among charities in the field.[2] In return for a grant equivalent to three years of salary and associated costs, for example, the charity would secure the appointment of a Macmillan nurse who would be in place for many, many years to come. There was good reason to think that Macmillan's donors, of whom there were several thousand, recognised and applauded the advantages of these deals.

Although Macmillan had played a very positive role in the growth of the voluntary hospices, in Henry Garnett's latter years, the relationship between the two had come under strain. This was because of Macmillan's growing influence in palliative care and the charity's emphasis on and preference for developing services within the NHS. Scott, even more so than Garnett, was committed to working with the NHS, and he made no secret of his opinion that the voluntary hospices had got it wrong, with too much emphasis on inpatient care. Scott was implacable in his view that the best way to improve the care of people with cancer was through the NHS and that the burgeoning hospice movement was a diversion. Now, the expansion of Macmillan, together with its modus operandi, added to this tension.

There were two causes for this. First, the Macmillan nurse had come to be seen by the public as an essential part of good palliative care for patients both in hospital and at home. There were some reports of patients and their families feeling thoroughly dissatisfied and let down if a Macmillan nursing service was not available to them. This was surely a good boost for Macmillan's continued expansion, but there were first-class palliative care nursing services that had not been funded by Macmillan and which, consequently, did not carry the Macmillan name. Many of these nursing services were operated by voluntary hospices, and they were displeased, to say the least, that their nursing services, as good as any Macmillan service, should be regarded in the public mind as second best. There were complaints that Macmillan nurses were set apart, and that they received, unfairly in relation to other palliative care nurses, the extra benefits of Macmillan-funded training and support. This problem was most recognisable when Macmillan and non-Macmillan palliative care nurses worked side by side. This was not infrequently the case in voluntary hospices, where Macmillan funds had often been sought at the beginning to establish a domiciliary nursing service, but where the hospice had added to it later from its own resources. There was no easy solution to this problem of identity. In several hospitals, non-Macmillan palliative care nurses were given licence to adopt the Macmillan name, and with this came access to Macmillan's nurse education programme.

However, this was not a solution that would find much favour with the voluntary hospices.

The second cause of the problem was money. Although Macmillan's funding commitment for a Macmillan nurse in a particular post ended after three years, local people of the area would often continue to give money to Macmillan year after year. As the number of Macmillan nurses expanded, so too did Macmillan's income from legacies. There was much evidence that it was the family and friends of patients cared for by Macmillan nurses who would then leave gifts to Macmillan in their own wills. Voluntary hospices looked on this with some disgruntlement, and in a few cases with outright resentment since, despite some financial support from the NHS, most of them had the ever arduous task of raising funds every year to pay their way.

There were claims that Macmillan's fund-raising publicity was unfair and that the charity raised money on a false premise. The problem was particularly acute in voluntary hospices with resident Macmillan nurse teams, because the hospice fund-raisers believed that any money raised for, or left to, Macmillan by patients, friends and relatives, or even the wider community, was money that was really meant for the hospice. It led to one or two hospices, including St Luke's Hospice in Sheffield with a long-time friendly association with Macmillan, removing the Macmillan name altogether from its domiciliary nurses. Some senior figures from the voluntary hospices called for the Macmillan name to be dropped from all Macmillan nurses and other services as soon as the Macmillan funding had expired. One or two others even proposed that Macmillan should stop all fund-raising activities in areas where there were voluntary hospices operating, even though these areas made up the greater part of the United Kingdom. They were calling, in effect, for Macmillan to shut up shop.

Macmillan's fund-raising publicity had always made it clear that its way of working was to pump-prime new Macmillan services, and that in return for its three or so years of funding, a new Macmillan nurse would be a permanent appointment. Of course, the ability of people to absorb the constant stream of information conveyed to them is limited, but far from being misled, there was reason to believe that the public was very much in favour of Macmillan's pump-priming association with the

NHS, which they thought was really rather smart. Local companies and businesses making donations to Macmillan saw it as shrewd, business-like thinking. The pump-priming model gave Macmillan, and those who donated to it, a long-term return on a limited investment or, to use a term from across the Atlantic, 'more bang for the buck'.

The changing dynamics of the National Health Service, and particularly the formation of NHS purchasers and providers, was an added stage for conflict. In 1991 a new national forum was set up to bring together all the organisations, voluntary and NHS, in the palliative care sector in England and Wales.[3] Named, rather long-windedly and pedantically, the National Council for Hospice and Specialist Palliative Care Services,[4] it was funded by a large grant from British Gas plc, and by smaller grants from Macmillan, Marie Curie and Help the Hospices. The council's role was to promote hospice and palliative care, and to improve its standards and availability. With a representative structure, although somewhat dominated by the voices of the voluntary hospices, the council was a good place for relationships and rivalries to be discussed, and they were on several occasions.

The crux of most of the troubles was the fear that Macmillan would instigate and support new palliative care services for an NHS provider which might be in competition with the palliative care services of a voluntary hospice. In theory this was quite possible, although Macmillan's policy was only to initiate new services that had the approval of, and the long-term funding commitment of, NHS purchasers. In fact, Scott thought that the need for competition for cancer services within the NHS was very doubtful and he had written saying so to the then Secretary of State for Health, Kenneth Clarke, back in 1989. But he also acknowledged that power within the NHS had shifted and that ultimately the new purchasers were going to have the final say. At the same time, the present Secretary of State for Health, Virginia Bottomley, had given the voluntary hospices new promises of financial support, and their funding position, though often variable, was rarely parlous.

The bottom line remained that Macmillan's policy was to improve palliative care within the hospitals, clinics and community services of the National Health Service, and this purpose was never going to be at one with the policy of the voluntary hospices. Scott's relationship with the council remained unhappy. Scott's successor, Nicholas Young, made a special effort to build stronger relations with the council. He took on the role of vice chairman of the council and always remained open to dialogue with voluntary hospices both individually and collectively. However, despite Young's far more emollient approach to the voluntary hospices, an element of tension always remained. It dissipated as the focus of Macmillan's work broadened and moved towards mainstream cancer care.

Some degree of rivalry among charities has always been present, and it is not necessarily a negative thing. Charities are no different from other organisations and they can become complacent and resistant to change or to new ideas. New charities are often needed to complement or even to challenge the work of others. The Cancer Research Campaign was, after all, founded as a rival to the Imperial Cancer Research Fund. In more recent times, the proliferation of charities in the field of, say, breast cancer or bowel cancer, is testimony to the myriad of approaches to cancer, its prevention, care and cure.

One of the factors that contributes to the charity sector being so vibrant is the relative ease with which new charities can be established and recognised by the statutory regulators. However, existing charities are rarely so sanguine about new ones being established in their area of interest. It was probably in Douglas Macmillan's mind in 1948 that the new Marie Curie Memorial Foundation was an unnecessary addition to the cancer care sector, and that its founders would have been much wiser to have thrown their lot in with Macmillan's Society. But whatever the arguments might have been some sixty years ago, the founders of the Marie Curie Memorial Foundation created a charity that has played a formidable role in both cancer research and care. Within a couple of years, the Foundation had overtaken the National Society for Cancer Relief as a builder and operator of hospices, and as the far more vigorous and innovative charity in the sector. It was not until Garnett, and then Scott, had pushed forward with the continuing care units and the Macmillan nurses, that the two charities began to approach some sort of parity. Some element of rivalry between the two charities has always been present because both organisations are so ambitious in their aspirations to fight cancer, but much of this rivalry has been among fund-raising staff and volunteers.

Over the years, Macmillan and Marie Curie had mostly gone their separate ways, and like two great ocean-going liners, had occasionally met up in port or passed at some distance at sea. Although the two charities had quite similar objectives, their respective trustees followed quite different courses. From its beginning, Marie Curie operated a scientific cancer research establishment so it was never exclusively a cancer care charity. The Marie Curie founders also decided that it would be a direct provider of cancer care services, and it began with developing the Marie Curie centres. These eleven Marie Curie centres or hospices, all large and mainly located in Britain's largest conurbations, were always run, directly, by the Foundation. They were, and still are, centres of excellence with teaching facilities, and with consultant medical staff who work closely with their colleagues in the local NHS hospitals. The Marie Curie hospices have always received some level of funding, variable with each, from the NHS. After its hospices were established, Marie Curie began its home nursing service. The Marie Curie nurses provide a night nursing service for patients at home who are close to death. In the somewhat clichéd, but nevertheless aptly descriptive, words, Marie Curie nurses are 'hands on' nurses. They provide bedside nursing to the gravely ill. The Marie Curie charity directly employs the Marie Curie nurses and manages the service to patients. The NHS makes a contribution to the costs of operating the service of less than 50 per cent when the overhead costs are taken into account. The other Marie Curie services are a major education and teaching programme, and a laboratory-type cancer research centre. Despite the work of the Macmillan and Marie Curie charities being different and complementary, there has long been some degree of confusion between them in the public mind, although it is not clear how great this is. Most potential for uncertainty, of course, has arisen from confusion between Macmillan nurses and Marie Curie nurses.

The expansion of palliative care and the leading roles of Macmillan and Marie Curie, coupled with the greater interest from government during the 1980s, encouraged much more formal and informal contact between the two charities. In 1985 Marie Curie had appointed as its director general Michael Carleton-Smith,[5] a retired major general. Scott and Carleton-Smith had been cadets at Sandhurst though they were not acquainted at the time. Both had strong personalities, and ambitions to match, and Carleton-Smith was as determined as Scott to push his organisation forward. This led to one or two instances of somewhat nugatory rivalry, such as when Carleton-Smith complained in 1988 about Macmillan's use of a strap-line, *Leading the Way in Cancer Care*, because it might imply that Macmillan was ahead of Marie Curie in the sector. Scott's explanation and justification, that the phrase was intended to refer to Macmillan's role in leading innovation, was probably not sufficient appeasement. In reality, Scott saw the Marie Curie charity in much the same way as he would have seen a rival company in business.

Of particular interest to Scott was the Marie Curie nurse, since it had the potential to become as powerful an icon as the Macmillan nurse, and therefore an equally powerful focus for fund-raising. Indeed, in the eyes of some, the Marie Curie nurse possibly had a much stronger image because of the 'hands on' nature of their work, which was far closer to the public image of what a nurse should do, and indeed what they had done since the days of Florence Nightingale. The concept of the highly trained and expert clinical nurse specialist, as the Macmillan nurse had become, was not easy for the traditionally minded public to take in. Moreover, the work of the Marie Curie nurse was crucial if patients really were to be given the opportunity to die at home, because it was at this often harrowing time that carers found it most difficult to cope.

Unfortunately, because of serious funding problems within the NHS, Marie Curie nurses were not always available to patients and families when they were most needed. Scott proposed a scheme whereby Macmillan would, through its patient welfare programme, offer to fund the NHS contribution for the service of a Marie Curie nurse on a case-by-case basis, where no other NHS funds were available or where NHS funding had run out. In this way, the supply of Marie Curie nursing services could be expanded to improve the extent of the cover available to patients. Scott remarked, quite rightly, that for Macmillan this was a much more cost-effective option than the alternative, which was Macmillan paying the full cost of a private nurse to care for the patient.

Accordingly, on 1 October 1992, Macmillan's Head of Patient Welfare, Neville Teller,[6] sent a notice to all NHS health authorities and trusts with this offer.

The reaction of Carleton-Smith and his colleagues to this gesture was, not surprisingly, one of some indignation, not least because the proposal had not first been discussed with them. This was, to be sure, an unnecessary discourtesy. Much more importantly, the initiative could have had major implications for Marie Curie's budgets, because every additional Marie Curie nurse service to a patient would trigger a request for Marie Curie to meet its half of the cost. Marie Curie just did not have the funds to meet an unexpectedly higher and unbudgeted demand for its nursing services. In response, Scott offered that Macmillan should make grants to fund the Marie Curie contribution to the service as well. This was a good offer and fully within Macmillan's way of working with other organisations to achieve better cancer services. It was not, however, an offer that Marie Curie could easily accept.

There were some practical problems, since Macmillan's patient grants were means tested, whereas Marie Curie nursing services were not, but these could probably have been worked through in discussion and negotiation. There was no further dialogue, though, with the result that the Macmillan scheme to support Marie Curie nurses was quietly dropped before it ever got off the ground. What the episode did do, more positively, was to draw attention to the potential for much greater collaboration between the two charities, and how, as a result, much more might be done for cancer patients. Scott, meanwhile, seriously considered the possibility of Macmillan setting up its own 'hands on' nursing service to fill the gaps that the Marie Curie nurses could not cover. The need for more open and serious discussions between the two charities was patently clear. These began about a year later.

Outright merger of the two charities was at first ruled out. The thinking was that closer collaboration and more day-to-day contact at all levels could lead to some formal partnership or even unity in the long term, but there was much to gain in the short term from greater cooperation. The first series of talks about closer cooperation began in December 1994 with six executives from each charity, but they excluded Scott and Carleton-Smith. They concluded that the most likely areas for greater working together were in the provision of palliative care education and training and joint fund-raising initiatives, and, probably most importantly, the nursing services. To these, Scott proposed to add the cancer buildings programme, the overseas programme, and even joining together the public affairs teams of the two charities. Scott also set out in a letter to Carleton-Smith[7] the crux of the difference of approaches adopted by Macmillan and Marie Curie. He said:

> We [Macmillan] are essentially facilitators, in the sense that we give grants to others to set up and run services … for a limited period of time. With the exception of Patient Grants, we provide nothing direct to the 'consumer'. You [Marie Curie] on the other hand are providers of a range of services direct to the patient.
>
> Whilst this is a fundamental difference in approach and philosophy, it actually makes it easier in many ways for us to work together. Our whole 'business' is facilitating providers. … With this background there is absolutely no reason why we should not facilitate services which would be provided by you. Indeed in the interests of seamlessness, comprehensiveness, integration and all those praiseworthy things, there is every reason why we should. … the facilitator/provider difference makes it difficult for us to merge, because we are not used to, and do not like, the heavy baggage train of long term commitments such as you have with the Marie Curie Centres. But collaboration and co-operation is another matter.

Scott's observations were manifest, as they were probably cardinal. The two charities were complementary in their approach and in what they did, but whether this implied that fusion was possible was a different matter.

All of the subsequent discussions were friendly and positive, although they tended to be about describing the charities' respective services rather than preparing clear plans for joint working. At the same time, more and more managers met with their opposite numbers and built up a closer rapport. Doubtless because of these constructive contacts, an impetus driving towards full merger began to develop, eventually shared enthusiastically by Scott and Carleton-Smith themselves. Moreover, the timing was apt. Scott was due to retire in June 1995, and Carleton-Smith the following year, so there would have been an opportunity for a new chief executive to be appointed to lead the project forward.

However, Scott's initial reservations to fully merge remained a fundamental point that had not been addressed. It was not clear whether a new merged charity would take the Macmillan role as a facilitator and developer, or the Marie Curie role as a service provider, or alternatively whether it could take on both roles. There was an underlying concern among some trustees and staff, in both charities, that merger would put at risk what each held most important for their charity's success.

It was Macmillan's Board which finally drew the merger discussions to a halt, but only in a way that kept open the possibility of greater working together in the future. The Board's resolution, agreed on 14 December 1994, was:

> to pursue with ... Marie Curie ... further discussions on how the two organisations might collaborate in providing services to people with cancer and their carers where that collaboration might lead to more effective and complementary service provision, but that there was no overall advantage to the two organisations merging together and that any discussions with that objective would cease.

Macmillan's need to appoint a new chief executive to succeed Scott meant that further exploratory talks were, in any event, not immediately feasible. On the other hand, Macmillan's chairman, Richard Hambro, thought that an opportunity had been missed, or at least that the matter deserved a much more thorough and considered thought. This was the brief that Hambro gave to Scott's successor Nicholas Young.

A year after Young's appointment, Marie Curie appointed Sir Nicholas Fenn to replace Carleton-Smith. Fenn was a retired diplomat who had served most recently as the British High Commissioner in India. He and Young soon built up a good working relationship, and some of the mistrust that had been a feature of the past was dispelled. In 1999 Macmillan agreed in principle to give financial support to the building of a new Marie Curie Centre in Bradford, a proposal somewhat reminiscent of when the Duchess of Roxburghe persuaded the Society to help pay for the new Marie Curie centre in Glasgow nearly forty years before.

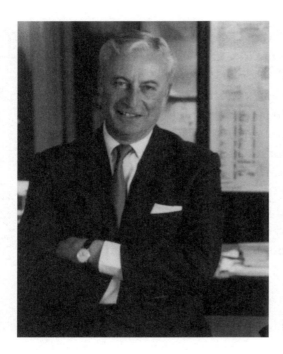

Richard Hambro.

This important gesture, among other things, led the following year to renewed discussions about a merger of the two charities. Young and Fenn, backed by their respective trustees, were enthusiastic about the advantages that merger might bring. They saw that the creation of a super-sized cancer care charity would bring all the internal benefits of economies of scale, while producing what would probably have been the most powerful force in the UK for improving cancer care. However, these discussions too were to founder, and this time it was Marie Curie's trustees who pulled back from any fateful decision. The reason was that Marie Curie's recent income had been below expectation and the charity's trustees wanted to focus their efforts on reversing this trend before any merger took place, otherwise they feared Marie Curie would enter into advanced negotiations as a weakened partner.[8]

Of course, Macmillan's most important relationship has not been with other charities, but with the National Health Service. This relationship has been the door to Macmillan's success from the 1970s onwards. For the many parts that make up the NHS, Macmillan has been a useful source of funds, and sometimes of expertise, which could be directed at improving cancer and palliative care services. All that was needed was agreement about what those new services should be. The health authorities and hospitals, and later the NHS trusts, welcomed Macmillan's participation because it would help them to achieve their objectives and priorities – and at an earlier date than would otherwise be possible. It is, however, worth not losing sight of Macmillan's spending within the overall perspective of the NHS. To use 1995 as the example, Macmillan spent nearly £21 million on cancer and palliative care services within the NHS. In the year 1995–96, the total expenditure of the NHS was more than £35 billion, so Macmillan's contribution was truly small by any comparison. Macmillan's strength has been rather the concentration of its funding on carefully selected projects that would have a major, but mostly local, impact. Between Macmillan and most, if not all, parts of the NHS concerned with cancer treatment and care there has developed mutual respect and goodwill which has only occasionally been strained. It is salutary to note that of the 3,000 or more Macmillan nurse posts created within the NHS since 1980, in only a handful of cases have those posts ceased to exist because of a refusal by the NHS to maintain them after Macmillan's pump-priming money had run out. This is testament to the value of the Macmillan nurses in the work they do and to a very effective working relationship between Macmillan and the NHS.

There have, of course, been problems from time to time. The widespread use of the Macmillan name within the NHS could have disadvantages for the charity as well as the obvious advantages. It has been argued by some inside the NHS (and also by some in the voluntary hospice world), that the name 'Macmillan' had really become a generic term, used to describe a particular type of care, and that the charity Macmillan could no longer claim exclusive ownership of it.[9] A number of NHS hospitals with Macmillan nursing services opened bank accounts in the name of their Macmillan nurses so that they could deposit donations by cheque, including sometimes quite large legacies. Often the funds in these accounts were used not to bring cancer patient care to an even higher level, but to fund the basic needs of the Macmillan service from filing cabinets and desks to computers. Wherever possible, Macmillan pushed or negotiated to have these accounts closed down, and for the funds to be used instead to support new Macmillan appeals or welfare grants for patients in the area. Success, though, was by no means universal. Ultimately the problem was not one of great importance, but all in all, a good amount of money has been involved.

A much greater danger brought about by the wide spread of the Macmillan name, at least potentially, has been the possibility that the charity might be blamed for the shortcomings of the NHS. A poor Macmillan nursing service, compromised by a lack of NHS funding, management failure or deficient integration with medical services, could damage the reputation of the charity as much as, or even more so than the reputation of the NHS. To maintain close contact with established Macmillan services, the charity appointed a number of nurse consultants who regularly reviewed the operation and effectiveness of each Macmillan nursing service, and worked with NHS managers to introduce any changes or improvements that were needed. Only in the rarest of circumstances did the outcome of a review lead to dispute.

The charity also adopted a practice of monitoring closely any complaints made by patients or families about Macmillan nurses or other Macmillan post-holders. Complaints, almost always from close relatives of a patient who had died and about the standard of his or her care, were uncommon, but they were usually highly charged with emotion and distress. Macmillan's interest was to be certain that any shortcomings in the service, or mistakes on the part of the post-holder, were put right for the future.

The friendly and constructive relationship between Macmillan and the NHS, good and successful for both parties, did still give Macmillan a dilemma. At its most simple, the question was to what extent Macmillan should publicly criticise the Department of Health or the NHS, or any of its constituent parts, for their perceived failures or weaknesses. Douglas Macmillan had founded the National Society for Cancer Relief, in part, as a campaigning organisation and he had been a frequent critic of government policy, or the inadequacy of it, towards cancer treatment and care. In the thirty years that followed Douglas Macmillan's retirement, this strand of work had rather been abandoned, by default if not by decision. Instead, Roxburghe, Garnett and Scott had been much more concerned about building new cancer and palliative care patient services, and latterly the NHS had become their chief partner.

From 1980 onwards, the NHS had become more and more a subject for the day-to-day squabble of Westminster party politics, and Douglas Scott in particular had no interest in becoming embroiled in that. Scott wanted to work with whatever government held office, and with whoever had been appointed Secretary of State. He was more than happy to express views and opinions about health policy and the condition of the NHS, but these would be in private to ministers, and not for public consumption. Even the word 'campaigning', when used in relationship to the NHS, had unfortunate connotations with protest and direct action, and would surely have attracted little enthusiasm from Macmillan's typically staid and spotlessly respectable members and supporters. On the other hand, Macmillan had become by the 1990s the cancer care charity in the UK with the widest scope and the widest reach, and with the greatest impact on the care of cancer patients. No other cancer charity had anything close to Macmillan's knowledge and experience of the cancer patient's journey from diagnosis, through consultations and treatments and more consultations, to final outcome. These were pretty compelling reasons why Macmillan ought to be more vocal, if that would lead to a better deal for patients.

Notes & References

1. Jean Gaffin, Chief Executive of the National Council for Hospice & Palliative Care Services 1991–99.
2. In fact, the Macmillan model has now been copied by others.
3. A similar organisation for Scotland had been established in 1989 – with Tom Scott being its chief architect.
4. It has since been renamed the National Council for Palliative Care.
5. Later, Sir Michael Carleton-Smith. Following retirement from Marie Curie in 1996, he became chairman of the Leicester Royal Infirmary NHS Trust. Like Scott, Carleton-Smith had close and personal experience of cancer.
6. Teller joined Macmillan in 1990, having previously been a civil servant at the Department of Health.
7. Letter dated 26 January 1995.

8. Marie Curie Cancer Care did indeed reverse the trend and in terms of income is a similar size to Macmillan. Fenn retired in 2000 and Tom Hughes-Hallett, a former banker, became chief executive.

9. St Bridget's Hospice on the Isle of Man unilaterally and with no consultation decided to call all of its domiciliary nurses, Macmillan nurses, although they had never been funded or supported by Macmillan.

17

Building on Success

Douglas Scott reached the age of retirement in 1995 following nine years of rapid growth and development. The charity had quadrupled in size over these years and it had come to occupy a leading role in the cancer care sector. He was awarded the OBE for his achievements. Garnett and then Scott would be hard acts to follow. The appointment of Nicholas Young in 1995, to succeed Douglas Scott as chief executive, was in many ways a palpable change. Young was quite different from his two predecessors. Aged just 43 when he got the job, Young had been moulded, in part, by the voluntary sector. He was educated at Wimbledon College and the University of Birmingham and began his working life as an articled clerk with the London law firm, Freshfields. He qualified as a solicitor and moved to a firm in Ipswich, Suffolk, where he came to do legal work for Baroness Ryder of Warsaw[1] and the charity she founded, the Sue Ryder Foundation.

The Foundation built or refurbished, and then operated, homes for the very sick and disabled, and also homes for the terminally ill. In 1985 Ryder proposed that Young should work full time for the Foundation,

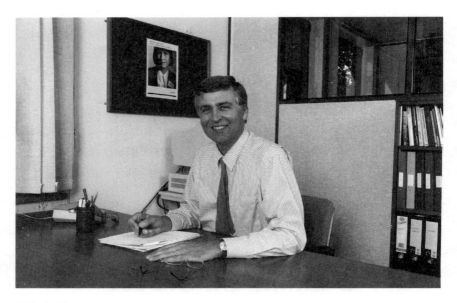

Nicholas Young.

and she offered him the post of Secretary for Development. Young
had decided that a career in law was not for him and that he could
achieve more, and gain more personal satisfaction, working for charity.
He accepted Ryder's offer and spent the next five years leading the
Foundation's programme of developing new homes. In 1990 he moved to
the Red Cross as Director of UK Operations, where he rationalised and
strengthened the range of emergency services available at home. Richard
Hambro, who chaired the Macmillan selection panel, saw Young, with
his legal background, as a 'safe pair of hands',[2] expecting that a period
of consolidation would be needed to follow the growth spurt of the
previous few years. Although much less volatile, Young was as ambitious
as Douglas Scott, and as determined both to make a mark on Macmillan
and to ensure that Macmillan would make a mark in its world. Young
was restlessly hardworking with spades of enthusiasm, and he constantly
sought new challenges and new horizons for the organisation and for
himself. He was also naturally boyish, kind and generous. Young's style
was to lead by achieving consensus and 'buy in' for his ideas. But he
could be forceful when required, and when engaged on a particular
scheme he would be determined and rarely deflected.[3]

Young joined Macmillan just as cancer treatment and care was beginning to take another move forward. He could see that there were opportunities to be grasped. Young had high aspirations for Macmillan and, from the beginning, wanted to give the organisation a vision of the future, or a clear statement of the organisation's dream. Douglas Macmillan had set out his own dream some sixty-five years before. The adoption of statements of vision and mission were becoming common practice in charities, and indeed in other sorts of organisations. They were means by which everyone associated with the organisation could unite around a common purpose. The idea of a vision for the charity, and what it might say, was discussed widely among staff and volunteers, but it was Anthony Simonds-Gooding who conceived the sentence that aptly described the charity's grandest ambitions. Simonds-Gooding wrote:

> Imagine a time when every person in the land has equal and ready access to the best information, treatment and care for cancer and where unnecessary levels of fear are put aside. Macmillan … dedicates itself to working with others to turn this vision into everyone's reality.

Douglas Macmillan could not have put it better.

When it was founded in 1947, there was good reason to suppose that the British health service was the best in the world. Providing a pretty comprehensive range of high-quality medical and nursing services to the whole of the population, and all funded out of taxation, was indeed exceptional. Many countries in Europe were, out of necessity, giving the highest priority to postwar economic reconstruction, and not to their health care systems. For the next four or more decades, the sick of the United Kingdom, with memories of the woefully inadequate pre-war health services, raised their voices in praise of the National Health Service, and they were uncomplainingly grateful for care they received, even when it fell short of expectations. However, as years passed by, there was a growing awareness that the NHS might not, after all, be giving patients the best possible treatment and care. This was backed by comparative evidence from other countries, as well as by the day-to-day experience of people using NHS services. Cancer was one area of particular concern, fuelled particularly by comparisons of survival rates from other countries.

The crude figures were worrying. During the 1980s and early '90s, the death rate from cancer was higher in the UK than in almost any other developed country, with the exception of New Zealand. The United States, Canada, Australia and most European countries all had lower rates of cancer deaths, and sometimes markedly so. But more significantly, the rate of survival for five years after a diagnosis of cancer was lower in Britain than in these other countries, including New Zealand, indicating perhaps that the treatment available in the UK was less effective than the treatment available elsewhere. Worse, for the commonest solid cancers that afflict mankind – lung, breast, colon and prostate – Scotland had the lowest survival rate of all countries used in the comparison, including New Zealand, followed by England.

Of course, care is needed when such statistics are compared. The methodology for the collection and analysis of mortality data varies greatly from one country to another and direct comparison may not always be possible. Causes of death are not always accurately recorded. Moreover, the success in treating cancer is dependent on many factors including, most importantly, early diagnosis. If patients are reluctant to report their symptoms early for fear of cancer, for which in the UK there was some evidence, then rates of cure will inevitably be lower than might otherwise be the case. But it was unlikely that extraneous factors alone could explain Britain's comparably poor record. It was as likely that there were some causative factors within the health system. There was yet another aspect to the UK statistics. They showed marked variations in cancer treatments and survival between one part of the country and another. Such differences were soon given the sobriquet of the 'post code lottery'.

Three months before Young moved into the chief executive's office, the Department of Health published the report of an Expert Advisory Group on Cancer, called *A Framework for Commissioning Cancer Services*. The expert advisory group was led by the Chief Medical Officer for England, Dr Kenneth Calman,[4] and the Chief Medical Officer for Wales, Dr Deirdre Hine.[5] The document became known colloquially as the Calman-Hine report. The report was of major strategic significance and it set the scene for the future development of cancer services within the NHS for the next decade. The report recognised, and rightly criticised, that the recent improvements in cancer diagnosis and treatments, and in palliative care, were just not reaching all patients in the National Health Service. Something was going wrong, and part of the explanation appeared to be that the treatment of individual patients was often not optimal. The effectiveness of treatment might vary from one hospital to another, or from one doctor or surgeon to another. The best cancer treatment and care was given in hospitals or by clinicians with the greatest skills and expertise in the discipline. The report recommended that all cancer services should be reviewed and restructured. The report said that the first general principle for the provision of cancer services within the NHS had to be that,

> All patients should have access to a uniformly high quality of care in the community or hospital wherever they may live to ensure maximum possible cure rates and the best quality of life. ...

To move towards this ideal, the report proposed a new three-tier structure for cancer services. At the base would be the primary care teams, based on general practice, and where of course a patient with cancer was most likely to go at first for medical consultation because of unusual or unexplained symptoms. The next tier consisted of designated cancer units, followed on top by designated cancer centres. Designated cancer units would be based mainly in the local district hospitals and would have to have 'sufficient expertise and facilities to manage the commoner cancers'.

Designated cancer centres would also be able to deal with the commoner cancers, but also the 'less common cancers [referred by] cancer units. They [would as well] provide specialist diagnostic and therapeutic techniques including radiotherapy.'

The report emphasised the importance of cancer units handling a sufficient number of cases of the commoner cancers each year for them to be regarded as specialist in that treatment, and also that medical and surgical consultants should each handle a sufficient number of those cases to give them sub-specialist expertise. For the cancer centres, it was important that they would have 'a high degree of specialisation and comprehensive provision of all the facets of cancer care necessary in modern cancer management'. In short, Calman and Hine were proposing a major shake-up of cancer services.

A patient with symptoms that might be cancer would be referred by his or her GP to the cancer unit based at a local hospital. If it was one of the commoner cancers it might be treated there, so long as the unit, and importantly its medical or surgical staff, had sufficient expertise in this form of cancer. However, more complex cancers and the rarer cancers would be referred on to the cancer centre where much more expertise was available. The greatest emphasis was put on specialisation, and creating NHS structures which allowed a patient's cancer always to be treated by a physician or surgeon of sufficient knowledge and experience. The report also gave emphasis to the importance of patient-centred and palliative care; of patients being involved with decisions about the choices of treatments, receiving better information and better communication between patient and professional carer. This was a report of very major significance and ambition, aimed no less than at shifting the UK higher up the international league table for successful cancer treatment and good cancer care.

So many aspects of the Calman-Hine report had echoes in Macmillan's own work. The charity had long been striving to improve cancer care and palliative care throughout the National Health Service at every level; it had been pushing ahead with projects to expand cancer information services, its Macmillan nurses had often filled the communications gap, and its medical programme had been focused on improving cancer and palliative care education for both hospital-based doctors and GPs. In his last annual report Douglas Scott said of the Calman-Hine report that,

> The key principles outlined in the document reflect Macmillan's approach to cancer exactly. ... This approach is at the heart of everything we do and is manifested through the many faces of Macmillan. ...

It was the Conservative government of the day that had commissioned the Calman-Hine report, and the government now endorsed its recommendations. Nicholas Young was quick to grasp the significance of the report and the greater role that Macmillan could play in improving cancer services. It would be Macmillan's strategy 'to link development of our work most closely with the Calman-Hine Report, giving priority to projects which are in line with it, and where the needs are greatest'.[6]

The government's acceptance of the Calman-Hine recommendations did not mean that additional financial resources would be made available to implement them. On the contrary, there was to be no extra funding, and because of this, little progress on implementation was made before the general election of 1997. However, with the Calman-Hine report in the public arena, cancer treatment and care had become a part of the high politics of the NHS.

Susan Butler, now Macmillan's Director of Public Affairs, was eager for Macmillan to be more active in public campaigning for a better deal for patients, and an opportunity arose in October 1995 during Breast Cancer Awareness Week. Macmillan vigorously joined the campaign which brought together several charities, and helped to distribute the pink ribbons worn as a sign of greater awareness of the disease. Macmillan also published a set of minimum standards for the treatment and care of people[7] with breast cancer which was endorsed by the Department of Health. Macmillan's campaign then went further, and it published a report, extracted from statistics released by the Department of Health, that ranked NHS hospital trusts (as most *providers* had now become) in order of their performance against these minimum standards, and it named those trusts that were at the bottom end of the scale. The story was picked up by the *Daily Mirror*, the popular and strongly anti-Conservative newspaper, which reported that:

> Thousands of sufferers never see a cancer specialist and are cared for by doctors with little experience of the disease. Thousands face delays and long waiting lists for diagnosis and treatment. Thousands are treated with old, out of date equipment.

This story made some people in Macmillan uneasy. The problem was not that the *Mirror* article represented a stinging attack on the government's stewardship of the National Health Service. It was rather that Macmillan's report named, and shamed, the poor performing hospital trusts. Tom Scott,[8] now a member of the Macmillan Board, was concerned about the impact this would have on Macmillan's relations with the medical and nursing staff caring for cancer patients in those NHS hospitals at the bottom of the league. He feared that it would damage the trust and confidence, and the mutually beneficial partnership that Macmillan had built up with them. Even more importantly, Scott was worried about the affect the publicity would have on the morale of the patients undergoing treatment in the hospitals publicly criticised. It was bad enough to have cancer, but it was then a double blow to be told that the hospital treating you was not really up to the job. It was a very good example of the dilemma that the charity faced when it tried to play the dual role of partner and public critic of the NHS. Getting the balance right would never be easy. On the other hand, the campaign had been very effective, focusing public attention on the less than acceptable state of cancer treatment in the NHS. It led immediately to Harriet Harman,[9] then Labour's Shadow Health Secretary, pledging that a future Labour government would require all NHS trusts to adopt the minimum standards for the treatment and care of people with breast cancer.

Young and his colleagues had no interest in alienating individual hospitals, and they always tried to avoid overt public criticism of any one in particular. However, Macmillan continued to grasp opportunities to proselytise the need for better cancer services, and to join the political and professional intercourse about cancer and health care. One relatively recent development in the cancer care sector had been a growth in the number of charities whose key area of activity was campaigning for better services. The charities working for people with breast cancer had shown the way for others. At the same time, the Cancer Research Campaign, now led by an effervescent Scottish oncologist called Gordon McVie, was increasingly taking the lead in a public debate about the resources available for cancer care. Macmillan could not ignore these new factors and still retain the prominent position it had earned within the sector and among decision-makers and opinion-leaders. Young was determined, however, that Macmillan would be constructive and not negative in its campaigning.

For Macmillan, the most important aspect of cancer policy of the time was the implementation of those recommendations in the Calman-Hine report, and it began its own coordinated campaign to achieve this. At a political level, meetings were arranged with government health ministers and their shadows, and contact was made with back-bench MPs who had an interest in health matters. For the first time, in 1996, Macmillan organised meetings for delegates at the conferences of the major political parties. The party political temperature was rising with the certainty of a general election in 1997, and the equal certainty that the state of the NHS would be one of the big issues in the parties' campaigns. No opportunity was lost by Macmillan to call on leading politicians of all parties to pledge their support for strengthening cancer services on Calman-Hine principles. With the opinion polls strongly indicating a Labour victory, Young and Butler made a point of lobbying Chris Smith,[10] the new Shadow Health Secretary who had replaced Harman. This then led to Macmillan organising a meeting for Smith and his colleague Tessa Jowell MP with eleven leading oncologists, including Michael Richards[11] and Karol Sikora.[12] The doctors used this meeting to argue, forcefully, for a much more robust strategy from a new government if the challenge of cancer was to be faced.

This meeting paid dividends after the election of the new Labour government in June. Labour had made the condition of the NHS one of the most important issues in the election campaign and Labour was now pledged to make radical changes and improvements. The Calman-Hine plan was fully endorsed by the new government. Meanwhile, Macmillan continued to campaign vigorously for improvement to particular cancer services. A campaign about gynaecological cancers concentrated on making people more aware of the early symptoms of the diseases and the needs of patients who had them. This was followed by a campaign for better help for people with lung cancer, a group that had long been at a disadvantage because they were often blamed, because of their smoking habit, for their misfortune.[13] The campaign drew attention to what could be done to improve the remaining lives of lung cancer patients – it was still fatal in the vast majority of cases – and particularly to help them breathe more easily. The campaign was launched by Labour's first Secretary of State for Health, Frank Dobson.

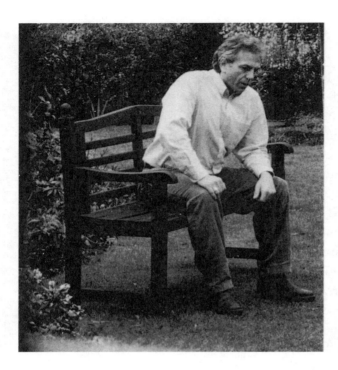

The lung cancer
campaign.

In due course, the Department of Health published a series of guidance documents aimed at improving treatments for cancers of the breast, colon and rectum, lung, stomach, and for gynaecological cancers. A Department of Health committee was also established to monitor the implementation of the Calman-Hine recommendations, and Macmillan's Director of Service Development, Dame Gillian Oliver,[14] was invited to become a member. Most significantly of all, in 2000, the *NHS Cancer Plan* was published, bringing together cancer prevention, diagnosis, treatment and care into a single strategy. Interestingly, it was the first time that a nationwide plan specifically for cancer treatment had been prepared since Walter Elliot's short-lived plan of 1939.

In his introduction to the plan, Alan Milburn, the new Secretary of State for Health,[15] admitted that 'decades of under-investment alongside outdated practices mean that survival rates for many of the major cancers lag behind the rest of Europe' and he ambitiously declared that 'this Cancer Plan sets out a programme of investment and reform to tackle these problems and deliver the fastest improving cancer services in Europe'.

Key elements of the plan were a continuing campaign to reduce smoking and improve diet, to establish targets for waiting times from referral to diagnosis and from diagnosis to treatment, improving the effectiveness of community services and the availability of palliative care, the better coordination of cancer services and specialist staff and improved training for practitioners. It was a ten-year plan with a target, through more prevention and better treatment, to cut by at least one-fifth the cancer mortality rate of those under 75 by the year 2010.

The Labour government was keen to work with cancer charities in implementing the Cancer Plan, and Nicholas Young, Gillian Oliver, and Macmillan's Chief Medical Officer, Dr Jane Maher,[16] had been consulted early in the plan's development. These discussions led to a new and novel scheme to appoint a cancer expert, called a Lead Cancer Clinician, in every Primary Care Trust.[17] These Lead Clinicians were there to play a strategic role within their trusts, developing and improving cancer services and providing a locus for information and coordination. Macmillan agreed to pledge up to £3 million a year to fund these new posts and to provide training and support for the post-holders.

The first Lead Clinicians took up their posts in 2001. Later evaluation of their role and effectiveness was particularly positive regarding the support that was given to the post-holders by Macmillan.[18] Perhaps not surprisingly, there was a strand of opinion in Macmillan that its campaigning work and its association with government initiatives was bringing the organisation too close to politics and to party politics at that. However, the chairman, Richard Hambro, had no doubt about the value of what had been achieved, and remarked that: 'It was important that politicians joined [Macmillan's] bandwagon, rather than [Macmillan] joined a political one.' There could be no doubt really that Macmillan had been helping to write the cancer agenda.

The Calman-Hine report and then the Cancer Plan brought a new focus to Macmillan's work. Hitherto, Macmillan's building programme had concentrated mostly on constructing inpatient and day hospices, essentially buildings for palliative and terminal care. Now, the Calman-Hine strategy gave the programme a new impetus within mainstream cancer treatment and care. Using the considerable skill and expertise that had been accumulated, Derek Spooner, and then his successor Simon

Henderson, set about developing within the NHS new buildings for cancer treatment. So many existing cancer facilities in the NHS were unsatisfactory. Some had been converted from Victorian infrastructure, even from old workhouse infirmaries, and they were cramped in space and institutional in character. Even more modern buildings could have an overly formal and clinical feel. Far from providing the atmosphere of safety and homeliness that would put patients and their families at ease, oncology departments of NHS hospitals could be pretty unfriendly places. As Diane Smith, a patient at the chemotherapy centre at Shrewsbury Hospital said: 'Such a dowdy place, so impersonal, you had to sit in a chair in the corridor with everyone walking in and out ... you just felt like a freak.'

One scheme, completed before the Calman-Hine report, was a refurbishment and extension of the oncology and radiotherapy facilities at the Western General Hospital in Edinburgh. Macmillan contributed to a building with an open and airy atmosphere with views across to the hilltop centre of Edinburgh – a world away from the low-ceilinged 'pre-fab' style building it replaced. The hospital had a catchment area for cancer services of about two million people, serving Lothian, Fife, the Borders, and Dumfries and Galloway. Jo Hockley, a Macmillan nurse based at the hospital said:

> The new building has created a completely different atmosphere. People may be feeling anxious and sometimes they will have travelled long distances for treatment. It makes a tremendous difference to have somewhere that feels welcoming and friendly. You just see people looking more relaxed.

The success in Edinburgh was a good foundation for many other schemes. The first was at Yeovil Hospital in Somerset where a small oncology suite was built and named the Douglas Macmillan Cancer Care Unit. It was formally opened in 1996 at a ceremony attended by Mrs Norah Hill, Douglas Macmillan's widow. This scheme was followed by the construction of two chemotherapy units, one at the Royal Lancaster Infirmary, a designated cancer centre in the Calman-Hine plan, and the other at Hinchingbrooke Hospital in Huntingdon, a designated cancer

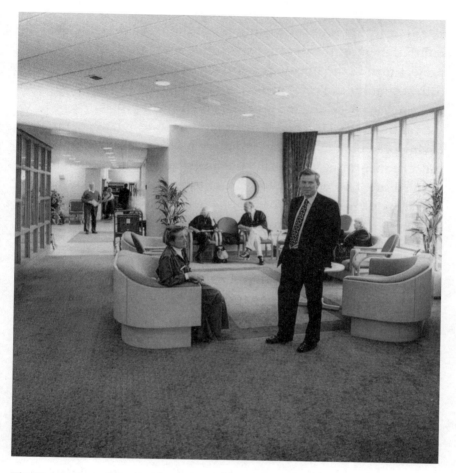

The Western General Hospital in Edinburgh – a world away from the low-ceilinged 'pre-fab'-style building it replaced.

unit under the plan. The late nineteenth-century buildings of the infirmary at Lancaster were impressive to visitors from the outside, but internally they left much to be desired. Patients attending the oncology department for chemotherapy often had to receive their treatment in the corridors or even in converted cupboard space. When working at full staff capacity the department was hopelessly overcrowded, making the administration of treatments difficult for patients and staff alike.

One of the consultant oncologists at the infirmary, Malcolm McIllmurray,[19] contacted Macmillan to see whether some help could be given to improve the facilities, and the result was a large-scale refurbishment of the department costing more than £800,000. The project turned the oncology department into a space designed for patient comfort and convenience. It was completed in 1997, paid for by a Macmillan appeal and the generosity of the local people.

Huntingdon's Hinchingbrooke Hospital was relatively modern, having been built in 1983, but it did not have adequate facilities for its cancer patients. So, Macmillan built a new and separate centre on the hospital site. This would allow cancer patients to go straight to their specially designed centre for treatment and care without needing to get through the hurly-burly of the main hospital. The new Woodlands Centre, as it was called, was opened by the prime minister, John Major, who was also the local Member of Parliament.

Over the next few years cancer treatment units were built at Poole, at Addenbrookes Hospital in Cambridge, at the Withington Hospital in Manchester, in Grimsby, Scarborough, Blackpool, Shrewsbury and in Halifax among other places. All of them were designed to make the experience of cancer treatment much less forbidding. Sian Dennison, a Macmillan nurse working at the Mustard Tree Centre at the Derriford Hospital in Plymouth said:

> People facing cancer are frightened when they go to a large impersonal hospital. The new cancer centre ... is a warm, welcoming, modern environment which has its own entrance and presents a friendly face.

Back in Scotland, a new chemotherapy department was created out of a former nuclear medicine unit at the Western General Hospital in Edinburgh, and in Glasgow a major refurbishment of the reception and waiting areas was undertaken at the Beatson Oncology Centre, the cancer wing of the Western Infirmary named after the famous nineteenth-century cancer physician of the city. The Prince of Wales came to officially open the much restored centre.

The development of cancer treatment centres did not mean that Macmillan's former emphasis on building palliative care infrastructure was neglected. On the contrary, palliative care was a priority for Calman-Hine and Macmillan continued to build inpatient hospices and day hospices both on the sites of NHS hospitals and in partnership with other charities. Macmillan's own team of experts worked closely with Jack Sinclair, Michael Barnett and other designers from the practice Architects Design Partnership, and with Christopher Burchell of the surveying firm Northcroft. This network of expertise was used to build day hospices in Liverpool, Ealing, Cambridge and Southend, to name a few, and inpatient hospices in Kirkcaldy and Brighton. The latter was a major scheme involving the construction of a hospice with eighteen beds and a day hospice on a new site in Hove. The Martlets Hospice, as it was called, replaced Copper Cliff, the home for people with cancer founded by supporters of the NSCR some thirty years before.

The greater focus on improving cancer services that was now filtering down through all integral parts of the National Health Service brought opportunities for many other innovations in Macmillan services. The number of Macmillan nurses continued to grow each year. By the end of 2000 there were more than 2,000 of them in post. Nearly 800 of these were Macmillan palliative care nurses working in the community, similar to those first appointed back in 1977. But the biggest expansion had been in Macmillan nurses working in NHS hospitals and those specialising in particular cancers or in particular aspects of cancer. Again, by the end of 2000 there were 413 of the former and 686 of the latter.

Most cancer diagnoses were given in hospital clinics, and almost all chemotherapy and other curative treatments were hospital based, and there was a self-evident need for hospital Macmillan nurses to be available to patients at these vulnerable times in their lives. Sandra Winterburn, a Macmillan nurse at the Norfolk and Norwich Hospital, explained:

When people come into hospital, they often feel vulnerable. ... It's a completely alien environment. As a Macmillan nurse, I have time to sit with them and talk to them about their anxieties. I try to bridge the gap between being a palliative care specialist who can answer any technical questions about the treatment they will be receiving, and being a fellow human being who genuinely cares about them and wants to understand what they're going through. This human contact is such an important aspect of my job; it's a powerful antidote to anxiety and fear.

The idea of a Macmillan nurse being close to a patient throughout the course of the disease was developed further with the appointment of the first Macmillan nurse attached to a GP practice. Tonia Dawson joined a practice in Dorset so that she could give support to patients even before there had been a formal diagnosis of cancer. As she said:

> The main ... benefit [of her appointment] is continuity of care. ... You can get involved right at the beginning and anticipate problems, linking community care to the often lonely business of hospital visits and treatment.

The influence of the Calman–Hine strategy also affected Macmillan's medical programme with the appointment of cancer experts to key positions from where their knowledge and expertise could spread. One example was the appointment of Dr David Farrugia as Macmillan Specialist Registrar in Urological Oncology at St Bartholomew's Hospital in London. The hospital was a cancer centre and Farrugia was an expert in bladder, prostate and testicular cancers. He explained that:

> We're giving more people access to specialist services because my work links services at Barts with local district hospitals. It's also a training post so it will help to develop expertise in this challenging clinical area.

Again, by the end of 2000 there were 257 Macmillan doctors in post, of which 77 were consultant-level physicians and 33 held teaching appointments. But it was probably in the area of primary care that Macmillan was able to make the greatest contribution, building on the work begun by Jennifer Raiman. There were nearly 100 GPs holding Macmillan appointments at the beginning of the new century, each of them working with their GP colleagues to improve the care of people living at home with their cancer. One was Dr Cath Dyer, Macmillan GP Facilitator in Cancer and Palliative Care for the Forth Valley Health Board in Scotland. After training as a GP, she spent ten years working at Strathcarron Hospice before she returned to general practice. As a Macmillan GP Facilitator, Dyer worked three sessions each week with other GPs, and also district nurses and health visitors, sharing with them her knowledge and expertise in palliative care.

Another GP Facilitator was Dr Keri Thomas, a general practitioner in Wakefield, who gave advice and support to GPs working in the areas of Calderdale and Kirklees in West Yorkshire. She developed the Gold Standards Framework for Community Palliative Care, a comprehensive collection of tools and resources designed to enable GPs to provide the best care for their patients. There were seven Gold Standards of care to which practitioners should aim, including the control of symptoms, good communications and the best care in the terminal stage. The programme to disseminate the Macmillan Gold Standards Framework widely to GP practices was led by Macmillan, before the NHS itself took on the responsibility.

There was another Macmillan service that was to grow and grow in the last few years of the twentieth century. The Calman–Hine report and the Cancer Plan put great emphasis on information. The Calman–Hine recommendations were clear that 'public and professional education to help the early recognition of symptoms and the availability of national screening programmes are vital parts of any comprehensive programme of cancer care' and that 'patients' families and carers should be given clear information and assistance in a form that they can understand about treatment options and outcomes available to them at all stages of treatment from diagnosis onwards'.

The Cancer Plan echoed these statements of policy. Macmillan had already pioneered local cancer information centres with the projects in Liverpool and Cinderford, and it had introduced the MAC Helpline for teenagers, so the charity was well placed to play a leading role in turning Whitehall strategy into good practice. Indeed, although cancer information services had not figured prominently in the charity's work for many decades, there had always been a constant stream of telephone and postal enquiries to Macmillan's offices up and down the country from people with cancer and their carers asking for information about the disease and the services that were available. This demand for information had already led to the production of the leaflet called *Help is There*, the directory of charities and other organisations providing cancer information and support services. In 1997 alone, 500,000 copies were distributed. Nevertheless, the directory itself would not eliminate the many telephone calls which had to be answered by someone with accurate knowledge and tact.

The solution was the introduction of the Macmillan Information Line. Using a freephone number the service started operating in December 1997. The service was not intended to provide callers with information about the symptoms of cancer or treatments, but rather it was described as a 'signposting' service, offering callers the information that was in the *Help is There* directory or information about Macmillan's own range of services. In its first twelve months the Information Line took 11,500 calls, and that number more than doubled by 2000. What made the Information Line particularly innovative was that it was staffed almost entirely by volunteers. Each volunteer had to be fully trained in the work and each might undertake to work a session every week, or every other week, and soon there were more than 100 volunteers available to cover the service. Although many thousands of volunteers had supported Macmillan over the years, they had mostly helped to raise funds. This was the first Macmillan service to rely on volunteers since the days of Douglas Macmillan, and it demonstrated again what great value volunteering can bring to charities. Nicholas Young was keen to encourage more and more volunteers into the organisation.

While the Information Line met an important need, the major thrust of Macmillan's new information services strategy had to be the development of information centres which people could attend in person. Catherine Dickens, who had previously worked for CancerBackup, was recruited as Head of Information Services to take this new strategy forward. Macmillan was able to offer to hospitals a comprehensive package of advice and resources to establish and operate cancer information services that would meet the criteria of the Cancer Plan. First, the Macmillan's buildings team could construct or refurbish a building on the hospital campus to accommodate the information centre, fit it out and furnish it. Second, Macmillan could fund, on its usual three-year basis, a centre manager, usually a Macmillan nurse or another healthcare professional. Third, Macmillan's Head of Volunteering, Richard Baldwin, could recruit and train local volunteers to work in the centre. Fourth, the Head of Information Services could provide protocols, manuals, consultancy and advice. The first Macmillan information centre was the Mustard Tree Centre at the Derriford Hospital. It opened in 1997. By the year 2000, information services had been provided at the hospitals in Guildford, Sidcup, Sutton Coldfield, Portsmouth, Liverpool and Epsom, and many others were under development.

Information centres based at hospitals were there primarily for the benefit of cancer patients attending the hospital for diagnosis of treatment, and of course their carers. However, the experience of the Macmillan Cancer Information Centre in Liverpool was that many of the callers were not patients or carers. They were instead people who wanted to know more about cancer, in particular more about its causes, how it could be prevented and what the early symptoms were.

It was quite impractical to have cancer information centres in all major towns and cities, but one way of providing this service was by using a mobile centre that could tour the country stopping at strategic locations. The first Mobile Macmillan Cancer Information Centre was commissioned in 2000 and began touring in 2001. Like other information services, the mobile centre made good use of local volunteers and the tours were planned to take in areas where there was a higher incidence of cancer. Several thousand members of the public called into the centre every year searching for more knowledge about cancer until this first vehicle was retired in 2008. It was replaced by several smaller vehicles making different tours so that more and more people would have the opportunity to use the service.

The new information services were supported by new leaflets and booklets about living with cancer, and trying to answer the questions that patients and carers most frequently asked. *The Cancer Guide* was first produced in 1997 by Macmillan and the BBC to coincide with a series of television and radio programmes about cancer. In the aftermath of the programmes, 23,000 copies of the guide were sent to people who rang the BBC helpline, and during the following year nearly a quarter of a million copies were distributed in all. *The Cancer Guide* has remained in print ever since. Other new publications have followed every year, so that today there are booklets of help and advice about advanced cancer, men's cancers, the care of the dying and about talking to children about cancer, to name a few.

Removing some of the fear and mystery surrounding cancer was a continuing theme in Macmillan during the closing decade of the twentieth century. It reached a high with the launch in 1999 of a new campaign called A Voice for Life. The idea behind the campaign was to give people with cancer the opportunity to put in their own words their experience of the illness, the impact it had had on them and how they were living with it. Their writings would help Macmillan and those treating and caring for patients to be more aware of their feelings and their needs. Their writings would also demonstrate to others that having cancer was something to talk about and that it did not have to cast an immovable shadow over all aspects of life. The campaign was launched by the Prince of Wales, who had become the charity's patron in succession to the Duchess of Kent. Speaking to more than 1,000 attending Macmillan's Annual General Meeting at Central Hall, Westminster on 23 June 1999, the Prince said:

> Tremendous progress has been made over the past 20 years in treating and caring for people with cancer – more people recover now; more people live for longer; and the quality of life has been improved dramatically.
>
> But what I find so distressing is that, despite this and despite the greater openness in talking about cancer today, we still use the same terrifying words and images to describe it. ...
>
> How many of us stop to think about the impact this has on people with cancer? From what they have told me, the reputation of the illness just adds to their suffering. It damages the quality of their life and it makes it even harder for the friends and family to cope. ...
>
> Through 'A Voice for Life' we want to transform the experience of cancer in this country. There has been so much talk about the problems of cancer. We must stop behaving as if we are powerless to change things. We can and we will.

These words were poignant and they must have rung familiar to many people in the audience. One Voice for Life, Kathryne O'Sullivan, said:

The last thing I want is for people to feel sorry for me. My first reaction was 'Shit' here we go. I wasn't devastated. I had seen my mum come through it at least four times. My chemotherapy was very strong. I'd throw up and spend a week on the couch. ... But I never gave up.

Another, Leslie Wood said:

You don't want it emblazoned on your chest, 'I've got cancer', but it's not a good thing to keep it secret either. ... You never anticipate it happening to you, but I'm philosophical.

David Matheson said of going to the day hospice in Ealing:

I'd hate to miss going. It's one of the highlights of the week. It's a very nice place. I do drawing, painting and talk to the people at the centre. Everyone is very kind. I've made friends there and we're always looking out for each other.

These Voices for Life and many like them reflected the day-to-day feelings and experience of ordinary people with cancer. They were positive and determined to live their lives.

All of this new activity needed money to sustain it, and Macmillan's income continued to rise. All of the schemes and activities that had been the day-to-day business of raising funds continued with a new determination. Douglas Scott had established a new post of Director of Fund-raising at the close of the Macmillan Nurse Appeal and John Abbott, a former businessman and Cambridge college appeal director, had been appointed to that post in 1992. He was succeeded in 1998 by Judy Beard who had directed fund-raising at the Red Cross and the Tate Gallery. Both directors had success in both consolidating and then building on the higher plateau of income brought about by the Macmillan Nurse Appeal.

Working with major companies had long been a very successful part of fund-raising, and Macmillan now had a team of fund-raisers who specialised in this. The list of companies supporting Macmillan grew and grew, and included many household names: both Homebase and B&Q

supported Macmillan; from the world of finance there was Barclays, Allied Dunbar and Scottish Provident; and from the motor industry, Ford, Suzuki and Rolls Royce. One remarkable achievement was the decision of Tesco to make Macmillan its charity of the year in 2000. Tesco and its generous shoppers raised over £2 million for Macmillan. Meanwhile, the World's Biggest Coffee Morning continued to attract more coffee drinkers every year. Many very generous gifts came from individuals. One, from property developer Robert Ogden,[20] paid for the building of a new cancer support centre at St James's Hospital in Leeds, and another, from Barrie Webb, built a new oncology department at the King George Hospital in Goodmayes, east London.

There were new fund-raising initiatives too. John Abbott managed to negotiate an arrangement with the organisers of the London Marathon that would give Macmillan a guaranteed number of places each year. Macmillan has had a major presence at the event ever since. Judy Beard was particularly keen to attract new people, and younger people, to join Macmillan's fund-raising activities. One event was called Hold Your Tongue and involved children at 200 primary schools being sponsored to remain silent for a certain period of time. It was a very popular event – particularly among parents and teachers. A new type of event altogether was sponsored challenges. Those ready to face a challenge had to undertake a gruelling event, often lasting several days, to raise funds for Macmillan. One of the first challenges was a 440km cycling and hiking challenge from Petra in Jordan to Massada in Israel, backed by Sir Ranulph Fiennes. Many similar events followed with each participant having to raise at least £2,000 on top of the costs of the journey. Most participants raised much more. One was Nicholas Young, who hiked across the Sahara Desert to raise funds for his charity.

Nicholas Young left Macmillan in the summer of 2001, after six imaginative and energetic years and having been knighted for his contribution to cancer care. He returned to the British Red Cross as its new chief executive. During Sir Nicholas Young's time, the charity had continued to grow at an astonishing rate. Income was up from £38.5 million in 1995 to more than £70 million in 2001 and Macmillan services were reaching more people with cancer than ever before. Perhaps just as importantly, Macmillan now had the ear of government in a way that it

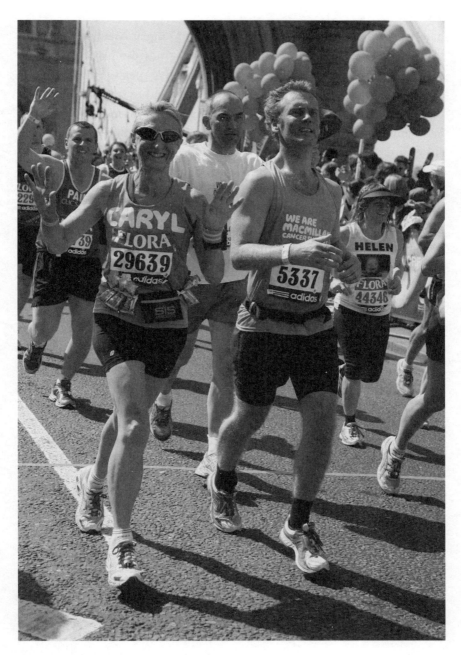

Marathon Runners, 2008.

had never had before, and to an extent that Douglas Macmillan and his friends could never have imagined. The charity was also playing a leading role in putting across to the public a less negative message about cancer, emphasising that it was possible to have cancer and to survive. Young had helped significantly to build on the work of Henry Garnett and Douglas Scott and he had run a happy ship. Young said that he always looked back at his time with the charity with great pride and affection.[21]

Young was not the only figure to leave Macmillan at this time. The chairman Richard Hambro had, by 2001, completed ten years of service in that position, and a further five as the treasurer and he thought it was time to step down. He had been a popular figure within the organisation. Always encouraging and always supportive to others, he had had an influence on the success of the charity that can be too easily underestimated. Young said that with his spirit of kindness and compassion Hambro had set the tone of the organisation.[22] His successor as chairman said of him:

> His contribution ... has been immeasurable. ... Under his Chairmanship the charity grew exponentially in resources, influence and ability to make a difference to people affected by cancer: his record speaks for itself.

In yet another example of cancer perversely striking those who have done so much to assuage the disease in others, Richard Hambro began his own battle with cancer in 2006.

Notes & References

1. Ryder was married to Group Captain Leonard Cheshire, the founder of the Cheshire Homes. He died in 1992 and she in 2000.
2. Conversation with author on 23 May 2005.
3. Young's first initiative was to invite his director colleagues to prepare a new four- to five-year corporate plan for the charity. Most of them were a little bemused, however, when for their first meeting he asked them to wear a hat that would represent their role within the organisation. He wore a baseball cap with the word 'boss' over the peak.

4. Later, Sir Kenneth Calman. He had been Professor of Oncology at the University of Glasgow and also a member of Macmillan's council during the 1980s. Following his retirement from the post of Chief Medical Officer in 1998, he became Vice Chancellor of the University of Durham. He also became a member of Macmillan's Board of Trustees.

5. Later, Dame Deirdre Hine.

6. Annual Review, 1996.

7. Breast cancer is usually thought to be a woman's disease and indeed 99 per cent of patients are women. However, about 250 men are diagnosed with the disease every year.

8. Tom Scott died of cancer in 1997 just days after reaching retirement age. He had made the care of people with cancer his vocation. A window to his memory is in the patients' reception at the Beatson Oncology Centre.

9. Following the election of a Labour government in 1997, Harriet Harman became Secretary of State for Social Security.

10. Now Lord Smith of Finsbury. In the event, Smith became Secretary of State for Culture, the Media and Sport.

11. Richards later became the first National Cancer Director or 'Cancer Tzar' at the Department of Health.

12. Sikora was at the time Professor of Cancer Medicine at Imperial College.

13. The work of the Roy Castle Lung Cancer Foundation, founded in memory of the popular entertainer who died of lung cancer brought about by passive smoking, has done much to change these attitudes.

14. Dame Gillian Oliver had been one of the NHS Regional Advisers in Palliative Care referred to in chapter 13. She was later Director of Patient Services at the Clatterbridge Centre for Oncology before joining Macmillan.

15. Milburn replaced Dobson in 1999.

16. Dr Jane Maher was simultaneously Consultant Clinical Oncologist at Mount Vernon Cancer Centre and later Professor of Cancer and Supportive Care at Hertfordshire University.

17. Primary Care Trusts were created in one of the Labour government's restructuring of the NHS. They were local bodies with responsibility for commissioning health services for their populations.

18. 'Early Days Yet' Evaluation of the Primary Care Lead Clinician (PCCL) Initiative, Centre for Research in Primary Care, University of Leeds, June 2004.

19. Later Professor of Biological Science at Lancaster University.

20. Later, Sir Robert Ogden.

21. Conversation with author on 22 September 2008.

22. Ibid.

18

So Much to Do

The new chairman, elected in 2001, was Jamie Dundas, the son of Hugh Dundas who had been chairman some ten years earlier. The younger Dundas had been a trustee of the charity for much of the intervening period. He was trained as a lawyer, but had built a very successful career as a banker and businessman. Although modest and unpretentious, Dundas had a highly intelligent and analytical mind which would penetrate most problems. His new chief executive was Peter Cardy who, like Sir Nicholas Young, had spent many years working in the charity sector. Cardy had been chief executive of the Multiple Sclerosis Society for some years, and before that, chief executive of the Motor Neurone Disease Association.

Shortly before he joined the organisation, the charity Cancerlink, which had been one of Macmillan's associated charities for many years, formally merged into Macmillan. Cancerlink had always been close to the several hundred cancer self-help groups that were established around the country, and so the merger brought these groups closer to Macmillan. This was fortuitous because Cardy's reputation was that of a

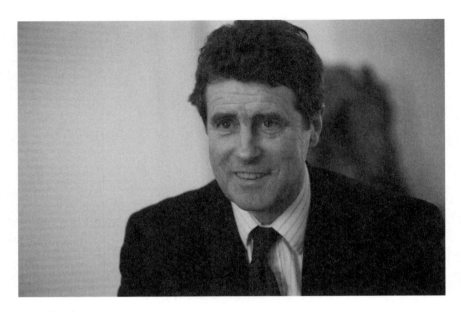

Jamie Dundas.

hard hitter, and not always a subtle one, for the interests of patients and carers, and this augured well for the campaigning work that followed over the next few years and for bringing the voice of those with cancer more to the heart of the organisation. Cardy was followed by Ciarán Devane, a business and management consultant who had been leading the life sciences practice for an international firm. Devane had a very personal commitment to the job because his wife Katy had died of cancer in 2003.

One other important post which should be mentioned is that of treasurer. Jonathan Asquith had been appointed treasurer in 1992 at the age of 36. Descended from the prime minister who had introduced state pensions, Asquith was a very senior figure in the City of London who brought considerable sagacity to the role. A keen cyclist, he also raised funds for the charity through sponsorship. He retired after ten years of distinguished oversight of Macmillan's finances. He was succeeded by Joseph MacHale, previously a senior executive in the US bank JP Morgan, and a director of the Royal Bank of Scotland.

★★★

One hundred years after the summons from King Edward VII to find a cure or a check for this 'terrible disease', progress had been both remarkable and disappointing. This was, and still is, a measure of the complexity of cancer and its genesis deep in the cells that are the building blocks of living things. Certainly, there was reason to be more hopeful than ever before that cancer would ultimately be conquered, or at least controlled. Although the number of people diagnosed each year with cancer continued to increase, treatments were becoming more effective. In the last thirty years of the twentieth century the incidence of cancer increased by nearly one-third, so that by 2000 there were about 200,000 new cases in England reported each year. Despite this gloomy statistic, the number of people dying from the disease actually fell by 12 per cent over the same period.[1] Since cancer is more commonly a disease of the later years, the increase in the number of cases had much to do with the ageing population of the UK. The more positive indicator of lower cancer mortality was due to a combination of screening for cancer and therefore of earlier diagnosis, to better diagnostic techniques and to new and more effective treatments.

Screening for breast cancer by mammogram began in 1988 following the recommendations of the Forrest Report.[2] The programme screened about 1.5 million women between the ages of 50 and 70 each year. According to the Department of Health, the programme detected in its first twenty years around 100,000 cases of undiagnosed cancer, and it was saving 1,400 lives each year.[3] Screening for cancerous or pre-cancerous abnormalities of the cervix as a national programme also began in 1988, although it had been available more than twenty years earlier. The programme screened women between the ages of 25 and 64 with as many as four million women tested each year. According to the Department of Health, by 2008 around 400,000 cervical abnormalities in patients had been detected and treatments offered. The programme accounted for the death rate from cervical cancer falling by 7 per cent per annum. In 2006 screening for colo-rectal cancers began for those aged 60 to 69. These cancers accounted for 16,000 deaths a year and together were the third most common cancer. Screening allows for cancer to be detected long before it causes any physical symptoms, making it much more susceptible to curative treatments.

Breast screening made use of advanced X-ray machines, and other technology aided the diagnosis and treatment of cancer by pin-pointing even more precisely the location of fast-multiplying cancer cells in the body. During the 1950s the cytoanalyser was invented, which scanned cells and differentiated the normal from the abnormal ones. Ten years later, Godfrey Hounsfield, a computer engineer at the British company EMI, developed an X-ray system that would allow doctors to see body organs and cancers within them in three-dimensional form. The system was called computerised axial tomography, or for short CAT, or just CT. Later still, magnetic resonance imaging, or MRI, was developed by Raymond Damadian, a US doctor and scientist. This quite different technology was based on the discovery that hydrogen atoms in the body resonate when they are hit by powerful magnetic beams. Both CAT and MRI scanning equipment use computer imaging to build an exact picture of the tumour, and thereby provide detailed information to the surgeon or radiotherapist about its position, size and shape. From just a handful of machines installed in NHS hospitals in the early 1980s, they became essential equipment. But they were also costly pieces of machinery with each costing £1 million or more with installation. It was very common for NHS hospitals to launch their own appeals for funds for the purchase of CAT and MRI scanners, and hundreds were in use by the end of the century.

As well as better methods of diagnosis, advancing technology brought about major improvements in treatments. The early radiotherapy machines did not show the promise that was expected. Only a small percentage of the rays from the equipment penetrated far into the body, so while they were effective for cancers on, or just beneath, the skin, they did not work for deeper-lying cancers unless they were given in huge doses. The invention of the linear accelerator, or LINAC machine in the 1960s, enabled the dose of rays to be directed deep into the body. More recent refinements, using computerised systems, allow high doses of rays to be delivered precisely to the shape of the tumour, so that the surrounding non-cancerous tissue is not damaged. Similarly, imaging technology helped the surgeon to remove more precisely the whole of the cancer and not leave malignant cells at its margin.

In fact, from the time of Christian Billroth, surgery had been the most effective treatment for cancer, and particularly if the cancer was discovered in its early stages. The better diagnostic techniques brought about the opportunity for more potentially curative surgical procedures. Surgeons, and particularly those that specialised in specific cancers, also improved their operating techniques. For example, the British surgeon William Heald pioneered the procedure of total mesorectal excision for bowel cancer, an operation which improved both life expectancy and the quality of life of patients. Surgeons specialising in the treatment of breast cancer learned that the excision of the cancerous lump followed by precision radiotherapy was as effective as the disfiguring mastectomy that had been standard practice until 1990. Keyhole surgery allowed some operations to remove cancer to become minimally invasive, and so much reducing the period needed for recovery, and the introduction of robotic surgery promised even greater accuracy and competence than even the most skilled of surgeons. The effectiveness of surgery was further enhanced if it was combined with radiotherapy or chemotherapy, either before surgery, to shrink the size of the tumour, or after surgery, to mop up any missed cancer cells.

Chemotherapy treatments had also been refined and improved, and in some cases were offering long-term remission or even cure. Many childhood cancers had become curable, and indeed were cured. Other cancers, such as multiple myeloma, could go into remission for many years. In the thirty or so years since 1970 there had been some remarkable successes. Karol Sikora recalled:[4]

> There was often a feeling there was nothing we could do. I remember a patient with testicular cancer, whose chest had become filled with metastases. A colleague asked me what we should do. It was straight-forward – nothing, just send him home to die. Ten years later, we would have cured him.

By using a particular combination of chemotherapy drugs, testicular cancer became curable in almost all cases, even after it had spread to other parts of the body.

Along with these improvements in cancer treatment, scientists were understanding much more about the biology of cancer. All cancers are triggered by damage to one or more genes, the units of DNA, the material that is found deep in living cells and which contains the instructions to build and maintain the body. These damaged, or mutant, genes cause the cells to divide uncontrollably, and this new growth, or neoplasm, takes on a quite different character from its original form. For example, genes in cells of a lung that have been damaged by smoking cause these lung cells to grow into a cancer which no longer serves any purpose in breathing. On the contrary, the lung cancer invades good lung tissue and ultimately makes breathing difficult.

The human body has many thousands of genes, some of which are oncogenes, which promote the growth of cells, and some are tumour suppressor genes which prevent the uncontrolled proliferation of cells. The corruption of either type of gene, or of both, can lead to cancer, and this explained why cancer tended to be a disease of ageing – the older a person, the more the damage to his or her DNA that has accumulated. The basic structure of DNA was discovered by Francis Crick and James Watson in 1953 and this was followed by scientists searching for an understanding of the bio-chemical processes at work and then for the precise genes, or mutations of them, that were responsible for particular diseases. The human genome project, finished in 2003, mapped for the first time the complete genetic material within human cells, and the cancer genome project, still under way, seeks to discover the variations and mutations to this genetic material that lead to cancer. This was research of truly awesome proportion. There are 25,000 genes in human DNA. Two of the genes that are known to be linked with breast cancer and also some other cancers, BRCA1 and BRCA2, between them have more than 1,000 possible mutations that can lead to cancer developing. Nevertheless, this new dimension of research brought with it the potential for new treatments to repair damaged DNA or to counteract its carcinogenic properties.

One cancer treatment that arose from this better understanding of cancer biology was immunotherapy, so called because it used synthetic antibodies that copied the action of the body's own defence mechanisms against cancer. The drug herceptin, used in some cases of breast cancer, is a good example. It sticks to the proteins produced by the cancer cells which encourage further growth and effectively neutralises them. Herceptin is effective for about 20 per cent of women whose breast cancer is caused by this particular gene mutation. Interferon is another immunotherapy drug used to treat several cancers, and avastin, one introduced for the treatment of bowel cancer.

Another biological cancer treatment was hormone therapy. The recognition that oestrogen was linked to breast cancer led to treatment with tamoxifen, an oestrogen blocker; and anti-androgens or anti-testosterone drugs are used for prostate cancer. Yet another new class of drugs were angiogenesis inhibitors, agents that caused the blood supply to tumours to be cut off, and of which the best known is thalidomide. Perhaps most exciting of all was the beginning of gene therapy, new treatments that sought to repair or alter the damaged genes themselves.

For Macmillan, these advances in the treatment of cancer, and the further advances that were likely to come in the first two decades or so of the new century, had several implications. First, it was clear that the number of people being diagnosed with cancer would continue to increase as the population continued to age. Second, it was likely that the number of people living with cancer would increase at an even higher rate as treatments became more effective and rates of survival increased. More people diagnosed with cancer would be cured completely, but many others would live for much longer with their cancers under control rather than cured. Sikora, again, predicted that for many patients, cancer would become a chronic rather than an acute illness. This was a different challenge, for it really did mean that people would need more support, and different kinds of support, to live with their cancer. All that Macmillan had been doing would still need to be done. More Macmillan nurses and doctors in hospitals and in the community would be needed to cope with the growing number of people with cancer, the best hospital facilities for patients would still be needed and the demand for the best cancer information would continue to grow. At the same time, the needs of the many people with terminal cancer would continue to be a particular focus, especially for those living at home. But helping people to live with cancer meant much more than just providing medical and nursing services. It could mean social care, financial support and many other aspects of well-being. Early in 2001, it was decided that greater emphasis should be given to these other needs, as well as the medical and nursing aspects of care.

The welfare of people with cancer and their families had been the primary work of the charity from the early 1920s until Douglas Macmillan's retirement more than forty years later, and it continued as an important strand of work. In 2000 grants amounting to more than £5 million were made to about 19,000 cancer patients in financial distress, and this figure increased to nearer £9 million in 2005. Mostly grants were given to patients who were living in some poverty, and this raised questions about the state benefits system and whether patients were receiving all that they were entitled to from the welfare state. It also posed questions about whether cancer patients were getting a good enough deal from the benefits system. In a report published in 2003, called *Unclaimed Millions*, the charity estimated that £126.5 million was being lost by 84,000 cancer patients from all parts of the UK in unclaimed benefits.[5]

There were really two points to the problem. The first was that so many patients just did not know about the range of benefits to which they were entitled. The second was that, wittingly or not, the state appeared to place so many impediments in the way of a successful claim. One patient, Lyndsey Baker, recounted her own experience:[6]

I was a mature student in my final semester when I was diagnosed with breast cancer. I'd been financing my studies with a student loan as well as three casual jobs, but I had to give up working when I started my chemotherapy.

When I tried to claim benefits from DWP [Department of Work & Pensions], I was told I wouldn't qualify for any help as I was a student. So I had to stop my studies and begin the process of applying for benefits which turned out to be more stressful than the cancer itself.

When I was at my lowest I had to spend hours filling out benefits forms ... then in the middle of my chemo requests for more information arrived saying that unless they received an immediate response my claim would be jeopardised.

It took eight months for any Housing Benefit to come through by which time I'd lost my home. In the end all I had was £55 a week in incapacity benefit.

Many other people, or their family members, had similar stories of frustration and distress to tell.

It was an obvious move for Macmillan to extend its own information services, including the telephone helpline, to cover advice about welfare benefits, and by 2005 it was a well-established service. A new Macmillan publication called *Help with the Cost of Cancer – a guide to benefits and financial help for people affected by cancer* was widely distributed to the information and advice centres. It also made sense to work with others to improve the number of services that were available at local level. One example was in West Dunbartonshire, once a shipbuilding town on the River Clyde with much higher than average rates of lung and stomach cancers. Three Macmillan-trained benefits advisers were appointed by the local council to visit patients at home and to help them complete the necessary claim forms. In just a few months, nearly £350,000 worth of state welfare benefits had been successfully claimed as a result of the project. Other schemes were established in association with local councils, particularly in those former industrial cities and towns with higher rates of cancer. It was estimated that by the end of 2006, these Macmillan initiatives together were helping people to claim more than £10 million in additional state benefits for which they qualified.

The experience of making financial grants to patients for more than eighty years meant that within Macmillan there was unique knowledge of the monetary costs of cancer that had to be borne by the patient or the patient's family. Of all the financial grants paid to patients each year, about half were to help with the costs of fuel, extra clothing and extra bedding – people with cancer will often feel the cold more. Extraordinarily, 5 per cent of grants were paid to help patients and their carers with the costs of attending hospital. The *Cost of Cancer* campaign and the *Better Deal* campaign were launched to make the government, legislators, NHS managers and the public at large, much more aware of the costs of having cancer and what could be done to mitigate some of these costs. The expense of attending hospital and hospital car

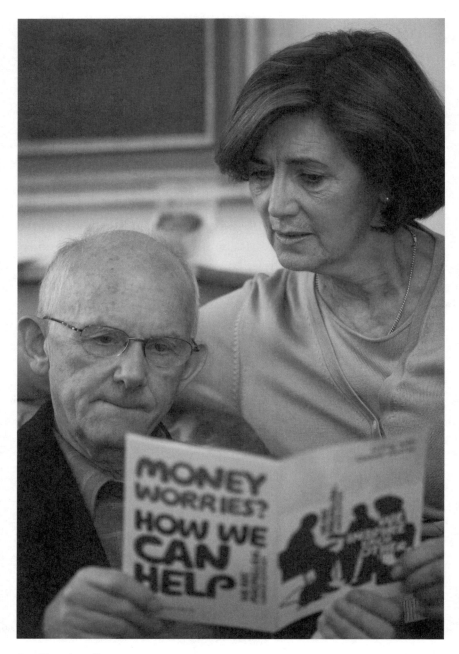

A guide to benefits.

parking charges were good examples. A survey of 1,200 people with cancer carried out in 2006, which asked them about the financial cost of their cancer, revealed that on average a patient made fifty-three trips to the hospital for treatment at a cost of £325. This was a significant amount of money to someone living on benefits or otherwise on a low income. Survey evidence also showed that the income of a cancer patient while undergoing treatment fell, on average, by 50 per cent. The Health Select Committee of the House of Commons recommended that patients should not be penalised in this way and NHS hospitals began to introduce schemes that allowed patients with cancer, and some other patients, to park without charge. The campaigns also focused on the cost of prescriptions, the higher costs of travel insurance and the appalling prospect faced by so many of the loss of employment.

These campaigns were followed, in 2007, by the *Working through Cancer* campaign. The focus of this new campaign was helping people with cancer to continue in work. Chief Executive Ciarán Devane explained that,

> About 90,000 people of working age are diagnosed with cancer each year in the UK. Growing numbers are surviving and many ... want to keep working or return to work after treatment. We know that employers want to help. ... I would like every workplace to understand what support they can give.

Most people had every intention of going back to work after cancer treatment, but it was not always easy. Returning to work after treatment was often not a straightforward matter and managers and work colleagues did not always know how to treat or talk to a colleague who had cancer. This new Macmillan campaign sought to give employers the support and advice they needed to help their employees with cancer get back to work. This was aided too by changes to the Disability Discrimination Act which from December 2005 included cancer in its definition of a disability.

The support that Macmillan was now giving to people with cancer was becoming more and more comprehensive. At the time of its merger with Macmillan, the charity Cancerlink had launched a major initiative

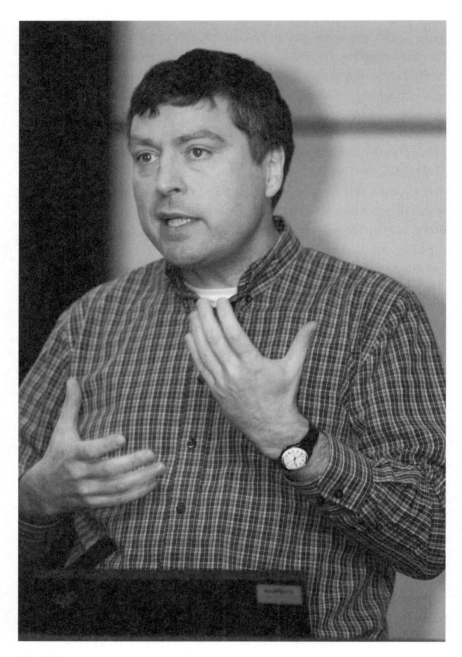

Ciarán Devane.

called Cancer VOICES. In some ways it was similar to the Macmillan campaign A Voice for Life. People with cancer had things to say – about what it was like to have cancer, about treatments, about the National Health Service, about public attitudes to cancer, about ways that things could be made better, and about so many other things. Cancer VOICES was the means by which those voices could be heard and it was embraced by Macmillan.

There were many elements in the Cancer VOICES programme. It could mean helping people with cancer to articulate their feelings and giving them the confidence to express their opinions. It could mean helping people to channel those feelings towards the media, or towards NHS managers able to bring about some change in the care of patients. It could mean Macmillan collecting the opinions and using them as part of a wider campaign, or as information that would lead to improvements in Macmillan services. One other important aspect of Cancer VOICES was the way in which it helped other people with cancer.

Self-help and mutual support among people with cancer had long been a way of helping patients to cope. A good example was the way a member of a laryngectomy club would visit someone having to undergo this surgery to give reassurance and confidence. Macmillan continued Cancerlink's work with the many support groups and encouraged the establishment of new groups. Macmillan's website allowed this mutual support to be put onto a different and much higher level with the launch in May 2006 of SHARE. This was an online forum into which anyone could place their blog about the way cancer was affecting them. Others might respond by talking of a similar experience, offering advice, or just by expressing empathy. Within a year, 100,000 people had visited SHARE to share their unique cancer experiences. Being able to tell your story and to know that it is familiar to so many others was comfort and support. The anonymity of a website allowed people who might otherwise be nervous of expressing their true feelings to speak openly. There is much in the adage that 'talking is the best medicine'.

One blog about the sleepless nights caused by worrying about a partner with cancer was viewed by more than half a million people and, incredibly, over 10,000 of them joined the discussion. Another, about caring for a dying mother, was viewed by 76,000 people of whom 447 responded. Some other blogs specifically asked for advice; 102 people responded to a question about getting travel insurance; and ten answers were posted about the side effects of the drug velcade as a treatment for multiple myeloma.

The development of Macmillan as the leading cancer support charity went one important step further in 2008 when there was a merger with CancerBackup, the highly effective and respected cancer information charity. It had a reputation for providing in-depth and accurate information of some quality and its list of publications included forty-four titles. Most of its patient contact was via its helpline, but 15,000 people each year visited one of their information centres. Astonishingly, 4 million people visited the CancerBackup website in the year 2006–7. CancerBackup had also been quite prominent in campaigning in the interests of patients and it provided the secretariat for the Parliamentary All Party Cancer Group. The merger between CancerBackup and Macmillan had a synergistic potential to create for the UK perhaps the best cancer information service in the world.

The development of Macmillan in the new century and the growth of its new services brought into focus Macmillan's public image, and posed questions about whether it was still right. The name of the charity had been changed in 1996 from the Cancer Relief Macmillan Fund to Macmillan Cancer Relief, but its logo was beginning to look dated. Other charities were now using bold letters and strong colours so that their publications would be noticed. Director of Fund-raising & Communications Judy Beard, and her colleague Amanda Bringans, led an encompassing review of how people saw Macmillan and it became clear that much needed to be done to change public perceptions. There was still confusion in the public mind between Macmillan, the charity, and the Macmillan nurses and there was still fear that Macmillan services were synonymous with terminal care. There was also doubt about whether the word 'Relief' was still appropriate. One patient said that 'It was the "Relief" that actually made me think, oh, this is the end of the line', and another said, 'You think that they're going to be giving you a lot of morphine'.

These comments were telling. Clearly Macmillan was not fulfilling its own ambition of helping people to live with their cancer if the image

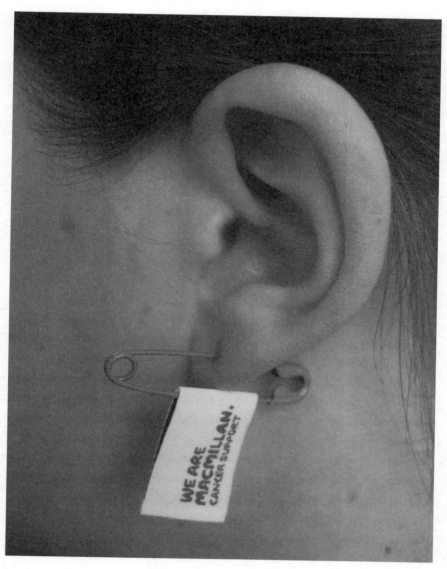

A new image and new style.

of the organisation, and indeed its very name, was putting them off. The words 'support for people with cancer' quite aptly described the very comprehensive range of services that Macmillan now supplied and so the name of the charity was changed to Macmillan Cancer Support. The official adoption of the new name was in 2005.

The change of name was accompanied by a new bold and assertive image and style. *We are Macmillan Cancer Support* was a new statement that could be used on any publication and in connection with any activity. The ambitious message behind the new image was that Macmillan was more than a cancer charity. It was a movement to improve the lives of everyone affected by cancer, and a movement that everyone could be a part of.

In 2007 Macmillan was one of the largest and most influential charities in the United Kingdom. Its income for that year was nearly £114 million. More than £7 million of that came from a single event, the World's Biggest Coffee Morning, which still held its place in the Guinness Book of Records as the largest participatory event ever. £40 million came from legacies left by those who were thankful for, or who wanted to remember, Macmillan's work, and much of the rest came from many thousands of individuals who, for one reason or another, wanted to give to Macmillan. By the end of 2007 there were 3,119 Macmillan nurses in post, 354 Macmillan doctors and 205 Macmillan cancer information workers. There were 74 carers schemes in operation, 87 benefits advice schemes and 68 static and mobile advice centres. During that year 333,000 people were helped by a Macmillan nurse, 62,000 people were cared for in Macmillan buildings, 128,000 attended advice and support centres, 24,000 people received a financial grant and there were 1.4 million visits to the Macmillan website. Macmillan was on target to have some contact with everyone who was living in Britain with cancer by the year 2010.

Douglas Macmillan would have been amazed. And he would have been very pleased.

Notes and References

1. The figures were different for men and women, with deaths of the former from cancer falling by 18 per cent, compared with deaths of the latter falling by 7 per cent. This discordance was due to smoking habits, with the postwar rise in smoking among women working through into cases of smoke-related cancers.

2. Report of the Working Group chaired by Sir Patrick Forrest, 1986.

3. *Screening for Breast Cancer in England: Past and Future*, Department of Health, 2006.

4. *Working Through Cancer*, supplement to *The Times*, 21 November 2007.

5. The research was carried out by the Centre for the Economics of Health at Bangor University and referred to the number of people with cancer entitled to, but not in receipt of, disability living allowance and attendance allowance.

6. Macmillan Annual Review, 2005.

Appendix I

Officers of Macmillan Cancer Support

Officers of the Society for the Prevention and Relief of Cancer,
1912–1924
Officers of the National Society for Cancer Relief, 1924–1990
Officers of Cancer Relief Macmillan Fund, 1990–1996
Officers of Macmillan Cancer Relief, 1997–2005
Officers of Macmillan Cancer Support since 2006

	Patron	President	Chairman	Vice Chairman	Treasurer	Secretary	Chief Officer or Chief Executive
1912		Dr Robert Bell	Charles Forward		W.G. Wilsher	Douglas Macmillan	
1914	Duchess of Hamilton (1)						
1915							
1925				Charles Forward			
1927		Countess Loreburn					
1931							
1933					T.A. Berry		
1934					F.G. Higgins		
1936		Constance, Duchess of Westminster					
1937			Major General Joseph Rimington	Douglas Macmillan			
1939							Reginald Gollop (2)

Year							
1940		The Princess Victoria Battenberg					
1942			Major General Lionel Dunsterville				
1946			Lord Darwen				
1949			Douglas Macmillan			Reginald Gollop	
1950		The Countess Mountbatten of Burma					
1951						Paul Steele	Paul Steele
1952					Dudley Chalk		
1953				W.B. Champion		Frank Georgeson	Frank Georgeson
1960							
1963		Douglas Macmillan	The Duchess of Roxburghe	Mrs Audrey Walker			
1964							
1966	The Duchess of Kent	Michael Sobell (3)				Gordon Tredwell (2)	Gordon Tredwell
1968				Mrs William Rollo			

Year					
1969			Peter Stanley		
1972	Henry Garnett (4)			Mrs William Rollo and Sir Charles Davis	
1973		Joan Bebbington (5)			
1974		Susan Porter (5)	Jocelyn Hambro	Sir Charles Davis and Peter Stanley	
1975		Tessa Scrope (5)	Lord Irwin		Mrs Jocelyn Hambro (6)
1977				Sir Charles Davis and Hugh Dundas	
1981		Joan Bebbington (5)	Earl of Halifax (7)	Sir Charles Davis, Hugh Dundas and Lady Margaret Tennant	
1982				Sir Charles Davis, Hugh Dundas, Lady Margaret Tennant and Mrs Richard Micklethwaite	
1983		Simon Cresswell		Lady Margaret Tennant and Mrs Richard Micklethwaite	Sir Charles Davis

Year							
1984		The Countess of Westmorland			Richard Hambro		
1985			Henry Garnett (8)				
1987						Douglas Scott	Douglas Scott (9)
1988			Sir Hugh Dundas			Christopher Seaman	
1989							
1991		The Marchioness of Zetland (10)	Richard Hambro (11)		Jamie Dundas		
1992					Jonathan Asquith	Paul Rossi	
1995							Nicholas Young (12)
1997	The Prince of Wales	The Duchess of Kent					
2001			Jamie Dundas				Peter Cardy
2002		The Countess of Halifax			Joseph MacHale		
2005						Victoria Benson	
2007							Ciarán Devane
2008						Chris Priestley	

Notes:

(1) The Society's report for 1913 describes the Society as being 'under the patronage' of the Duchess of Hamilton, but there is no record of her ever being actively associated with the Society's work.

(2) Reginal Gollop was appointed as appeals secretary in 1930. At the outbreak of war in 1939 he was appointed General Secretary and was the senior person at the Society's office. However, Macmillan remained in the post of Honorary Secretary. On the resignation of Lord Darwen as Chairman in 1949, Macmillan became Chairman and the post of Honorary Secretary ceased to exist. From this point, the post-holder of General Secretary became, de facto, the Chief Officer. The post was left vacant for ten years after Gordon Tredwell stood down.

(3) Later, Sir Michael Sobell; he was appointed President Emeritus in 1984.

(4) Henry Garnett was also appointed as Deputy Chairman.

(5) Joan Bebbington, Susan Porter and Miss T. Scrope held the post of Administrative Secretary; in the case of Joan Bebbington, together with the post of Relief Secretary from 1981.

(6) The Duchess of Roxburghe became Mrs Jocelyn Hambro on her marriage following the death of the duke.

(7) Lord Irwin succeeded to become the Earl of Halifax on the death of his father.

(8) Henry Garnett occupied the posts of Chairman and Chief Executive from 1985 to 1987.

(9) Douglas Scott was appointed as Secretary and Director in 1987, but his post was re-designated as Chief Executive in 1989.

(10) The Marchioness was appointed Deputy President in 1997 and held the post until 1998.

(11) Richard Hambro was appointed Deputy President in 2001.

(12) Later, Sir Nicholas Young.

Appendix II

A Chronology of Key Events in the History of Macmillan Cancer Support

1911	Death of William Macmillan from cancer. His son Douglas sets about founding a charity for the relief of cancer.
1912	The Society for the Prevention and Relief of Cancer holds its first annual meeting. Charles Forward elected chairman, and Douglas Macmillan secretary. Dr Robert Bell elected president. New Society committed to the anti-vivisection platform and proving the link between diet and cancer.
1913	Programme of cancer information and education begins with publication of booklets, leaflets and the *Journal of Cancer*.
1914	First World War begins and the activities of the Society collapse.
1923	British Empire Cancer Campaign is founded, and Society decides to concentrate its charitable work of relief.
1924	Society registers as a benevolent society under the Friendly Societies Acts. Society is renamed National Society for Cancer Relief.

1925	First grant to a patient recorded.
1926	Countess Loreburn becomes president.
1930	First employee, Reginald Gollop, is appointed, with responsibility to raise the Society's income.
1931	Patient welfare programme emerges and £80 paid in grants to patients. First attempt to open a home for cancer patients fails. Douglas Macmillan campaigns for more inpatient beds and other services for people with cancer.
1932	First full-time nurse visitors appointed to cover London and Middlesex, and York.
1934	Death of Charles Forward. First local committee established in Bath.
1935	Head office moves to 47 Victoria Street. Constance, Duchess of Westminster becomes president.
1937	Major General Joseph Rimington becomes chairman.
1938	Welfare payments to patients exceed £7,000. First grants made for patients to take convalescence breaks.
1939	Cancer Act passed by Parliament. Second World War begins.
1940	Princess Victoria Battenburg appointed president. Society's offices in Victoria are twice bombed and staff are evacuated to Cheam.
1941	First BBC radio appeal, made by the Bishop of Bristol, raises more than £7,000.
1942	Death of Joseph Rimington. Major General Lionel Dunsterville becomes chairman.
1943	Welfare payments to patients exceed £10,000.
1946	Office in Victoria re-opens, but patient welfare team remain in Cheam. Lionel Dunsterville dies, and Lord Darwen becomes chairman.
1948	National Health Service comes into being. Second BBC radio appeal, made by Revd Leslie Weatherhead.
1949	Lord Darwen resigns. Douglas Macmillan becomes chairman.
1950	Death of Princess Victoria Battenburg. The Countess Mountbatten of Burma becomes president. Reginald Gollop retires, and dies the following year.
1951	50th Anniversary. *Book of Cancer Relief* published by the Society.
1957	Margaret Macmillan dies.

1959	Third BBC radio appeal, made by Barbara Kelly.
1960	Society opens Helstonleigh in Southborough as a home for patients with cancer.
1963	Douglas Macmillan retires. The Duchess of Roxburghe becomes chairman.
1964	Helstonleigh is closed.
1965	The Duchess of Kent becomes patron and Sir Michael Sobell becomes president.
1966	Head office moves to 30 Dorset Square, Marylebone.
1967	Copper Cliff opens. St Christopher's Hospice opens.
1969	Death of Douglas Macmillan.
1971	Lillian Board Appeal launched.
1973	Macmillan home at Stoke-on-Trent opened.
1975	Henry Garnett becomes deputy chairman and chief executive. First Macmillan unit, at Christchurch Hospital, opened.
1976	Bing Crosby appears at London Palladium, and donates 50 per cent of fee to the Society. Sir Michael Sobell House in Oxford opened. Macmillan unit at King Edward VII Hospital in Midhurst opened. First Macmillan nurses appointed, at St Joseph's Hospice in Hackney.
1977	National appeal launched under chairmanship of John King.
1978	Macmillan service at Dorothy House Foundation in Bath started.
1980	Medical education programme begins.
1982	Second national appeal launched.
1984	The Countess of Westmorland becomes president. Charity re-named Cancer Relief Macmillan Fund.
1985	DHSS conference on terminal care opened by the Prince of Wales.
1986	75th Anniversary. Henry Garnett retires as chief executive and is succeeded by Douglas Scott. Head office moves to Britten Street, Chelsea.
1988	500th Macmillan nurse appointed.
1989	MACPAC programmes launched. *Help is There* is first published. Legal form of company limited by guarantee adopted.

1990	West Berkshire cancer day centres opened using Macmillan Green design.
1991	80th Anniversary. Richard Hambro becomes chairman in succession to Sir High Dundas. Launch of the Macmillan Nurse Appeal under patronage of the Prince of Wales.
1993	Macmillan Design Challenge. 1,000th Macmillan nurse appointed. First GP Facilitators appointed.
1994	Organisation decentralised into regions. MAC Helpline for teenagers launched. First carers' schemes begin in Stockport, Wakefield, Norwich and Solihull. First high-street Macmillan information centre opens in Liverpool.
1995	Calman–Hine report published. Douglas Scott retires and is succeeded by Nicholas Young. Breast Cancer Awareness week.
1996	Douglas Macmillan Unit in Yeovil opened. Charity re-named Macmillan Cancer Relief.
1997	Macmillan Information Line launched. *The Cancer Guide* published. The Prince of Wales becomes patron in succession to the Duchess of Kent. The Duchess of Kent becomes president.
1999	A Voice for Life launched by the Prince of Wales.
2000	*Cancer Plan* published. 2,000th Macmillan nurse appointed.
2001	Lead Cancer Clinicians appointed. Merger with CancerLink. Mobile information centre begins first tour. Richard Hambro retires as chairman and is succeeded by Jamie Dundas.
2003	Sir Nicholas Young leaves and is succeeded by Peter Cardy.
2005	Unclaimed Millions report published.
2006	Charity re-named Macmillan Cancer Support. SHARE launched on website.
2007	Income exceeds £100 million for the first time. Peter Cardy leaves and is succeeded by Ciarán Devane.
2008	Working through Cancer campaign launched. Merger with CancerBackup.

Index